Handbook of Positional Plagiocephaly

Satoshi Kusuda • Yasuo Aihara
Isao Kusakawa • Shigeharu Hosono
Editors

Handbook of Positional Plagiocephaly

JCMETS
Japan Cranial Medical Examination and Treatment Society

Springer

Editors
Satoshi Kusuda
Department of Pediatrics
Faculty of Medicine
Kyorin University
Mitaka, Tokyo, Japan

Isao Kusakawa
Baby's Head Reshaping Clinic
Chuo-ku, Tokyo, Japan

Yasuo Aihara
Department of Neurosurgery
Tokyo Women's Medical University
Shinjuku-ku, Tokyo, Japan

Shigeharu Hosono
Saitama Medical Center
Jichi Medical University
Saitama, Japan

ISBN 978-981-97-9163-7 ISBN 978-981-97-9164-4 (eBook)
https://doi.org/10.1007/978-981-97-9164-4

Based on a translation from the Japanese language edition:
Shouni no Zugai Kenshin Chiryo Handbook: Akachan no Atama no Katachi no Mikata, published by MEDICUS SHUPPAN, Publishers Co., Ltd. 2022.

This Springer imprint is published by the registered company Springer Nature Singapore Pte Ltd.
The registered company address is: 152 Beach Road, #21-01/04 Gateway East, Singapore 189721, Singapore

Preface

Medical care and medicine have a long history of maturation and construction based on the evidence obtained through the efforts of our predecessors. These discoveries will be passed down to future generations as "common sense." For those of us who are involved in medical care in this world and serve as communicators, we need the "courage" to take this evidence into our own hands, touch it, re-examine it from various angles, and verify it, instead of just passing it on from here to there.

The diagnosis of the head shape and size of newborns and infants holds a very important meaning for their subsequent growth and development. However, in Japan, there is no defined reference value for the diagnosis of cranial deformity, regardless of the presence or absence of the primary disease. From pathological cranial deformity to the diagnosis of positional cranial deformity triggered by orientation, pediatric medical practice, including infant health checkups, is currently chaotic over the diagnosis and correct choice of early treatment.

Are the discoveries and knowledge we have inherited as "common sense" really "common sense"? To explore this question, in 2020, we established the Japan Cranial Medical Examination and Treatment Society (JCMETS). This organization began its activities as a forum for discussing the health of children, who will be responsible for the future, from an academic point of view of "cranial checkups" (the details of the study group will be described later).

The positional cranial deformity is a multiplanar cranial deformity that can occur in infants both before and after birth. This, as is true of many other "non-closing cranial suture" head deformities described and reported in the literature, can lead to serious functional, neurological, and cosmetic ramifications and can have psychological consequences if left untreated. For example, pressure on muscles and nerves in the orbit causes sensory and movement disorders [1]. As a result, infants with cranial deformity may develop ocular and vestibular dysfunctions to compensate for the abnormal head orientation in space [2]. Moreover, considering that 85% of the skull growth is completed within the first year of life [3], early detection and treatment in this short period are of utmost importance [4].

Here, we provide an easy-to-understand handbook about the concept of cranial deformity, screening methods used in general infant health checkups, diagnosis in specialized medical institutions, and introduction to treatment methods. Also, there is a set of questions and answers to questions from families about cranial deformity and related papers that should be read are introduced. It is my earnest hope that this book will sublimate the "tradition" of the pathological condition of "cranial deformity" into a better medical "tradition."

Japan Cranial Health Examination Treatment Study Group.

Tokyo, Japan Satoshi Kusuda
Tokyo, Japan Yasuo Aihara
Tokyo, Japan Isao Kusakawa
Saitama, Japan Shigeharu Hosono
April 2022

References

1. Rekate HL. Occipital plagiocephaly: a critical review of the literature. J Neurosurg. 1998; 89(1):24–30.
2. Argenta LC, David LR, Wilson JA, et al. An increase in infant cranial deformity with sleeping position. J Craniofac Surg. 1996;7(1):5–11.
3. Aihara Y, Komatsu K, Dairoku H, et al. Cranial molding helmet therapy and establishment of practical criteria for management in Asian infant positional head deformity. Childs Nerv Syst. 2014;30(9):1499–509.
4. Graham JM Jr., Charman CE, Chaisson R, et al. Postnatal head deformation: anthropological observations and applications to the treatment of postnatal plagiocephaly. Proceedings of the Greenwood Genetic Center. 1988;7:156–59.

About the Japan Cranial Medical Examination and Treatment Society

The Japan Cranial Medical Examination and Treatment Society (JCMETS) is an academic research group established in October 2020.

In recent years, interest in cranial deformity in infants has increased, and some medical institutions have introduced treatment methods for cranial deformity in infants. However, there is no standardized diagnostic method for cranial deformity in infants. There is also a lack of knowledge among healthcare professionals about the natural history of infants with cranial deformities, and a standardized treatment for cranial deformities has not been established yet. In addition, there is considerable confusion in the field because the treatment of cranial deformity is not subject for reimbursement under the current health insurance system. In order to solve these current issues, this study group was established to promote academic research, train specialists in medical examinations and treatments, provide information to the public, and collect data on the long-term prognosis of cranial deformity in Japan.

Diagnosis and therapeutic intervention for cranial deformity are not necessarily a "one-to-one" relationship. This study group aims to establish an accurate concept of cranial deformity, initial screening for cranial deformity in infant health check-ups, professional diagnosis of cranial deformity, and appropriate selection of target population. The aim is to establish a system that can be implemented in Japan without delay. In addition, to achieve the purpose of the establishment of the study group as described above, the board members of the study group consist of multidisciplinary specialists, including neurosurgeons, pediatricians, obstetricians, pediatric surgeons, pediatric orthopedic surgeons, plastic surgeons, dental and oral surgeons, midwives, and physical therapists. In addition, general members who have many opportunities to be involved in cranial deformation in infants are widely invited to participate.

Presently, the most important activities are the dissemination of knowledge about cranial deformities in infants, standardization of diagnostic criteria, and treatment. At the first step, this handbook was co-authored by the core members of the study group. It is hoped that knowledge about cranial deformities in infants will be generalized, the appropriate screening will be carried out in infant health examinations, and more accurate diagnoses will be made at specialized medical institutions.

Accurate diagnosis of cranial deformity naturally makes it possible to implement appropriate interventions for cranial deformity. The dissemination of this book will be the first step toward achieving the purpose of establishing this study group.

《Website of the Japan Cranial Health Examination and Treatment Research Society》

https://www.jcmets.org/

Contents

Part I
Overview

Chapter 1
Overview of Cranial Deformity

Satoshi Kusuda

1 Definition/Incidence

An infant's skull does not comprise a single cranial bone as that of an adult's. It is made up of eight bones of six different types. Moreover, although these bones are fibrously sutured to one another, they are not synostosed as a single bone. Around the age of 2–3 years, the skull fuses as one bone.

In infancy, the skull is not fused because it is a period of rapid brain growth as a newborn's brain weighs 350–400 g, but it approximately doubles at 8 months of age and then reaches an adult brain weight of 1200–1400 g at 5–6 years of age. Therefore, external pressure easily displaces the position of skull bones, causing deformation of the entire skull. This is called positional cranial deformation.

Because there is no definitive diagnostic criteria for positional cranial deformity, the exact incidence is unknown. However, it was reported to occur in as high as 40–50% of infants in early infancy [1, 2]. In 1992, the American Academy of Pediatrics (AAP) recommended sleeping on the back for the prevention of sudden infant death syndrome (SIDS) [3]. Table 1.1 describes the recommendation for infant sleeping position issued by AAP at that time. Since then, people's attention has been paid carefully to the sleeping position of infants worldwide, and the frequency of SIDS has dramatically decreased, making it an important recommendation. However, cranial deformities have increased since the AAP recommendations [4]. Even if that is the case, it is obvious that sleeping on the back (supine) in infants must be strictly adhered to as a preventive measure against SIDS.

The frequency of these positional cranial deformities peaks at around 4 months of age and then partially improves with growth, with the frequency of cranial deformity reportedly decreasing to 3.3% at 2 years of age (Fig. 1.1) [5]. Positional cranial

S. Kusuda (✉)
Department of Pediatrics, Faculty of Medicine, Kyorin University, Tokyo, Japan
e-mail: kusuda-satoshi@nrnj.org

S. Kusuda et al. (eds.), *Handbook of Positional Plagiocephaly*,
https://doi.org/10.1007/978-981-97-9164-4_1

Table 1.1 Summary of American Academy of Pediatrics (AAP) recommendations for infant sleeping positions

• Several studies show a relationship between prone sleeping position and sudden infant death syndrome (SIDS)
• It is difficult to conduct a randomized clinical comparative study to prove the relationship between sleeping posture and SIDS
• Currently in the United States, it is customary to put infants to sleep in the prone position
Therefore, at present, there is a need to avoid the risk of SIDS
• Hence, it is recommended that infants with no health problems should be placed in the supine or side-lying position. (note: Excluding infants who require the prone position for medical reasons.)
Note: The American Academy of Pediatrics later dropped the side-lying recommendation

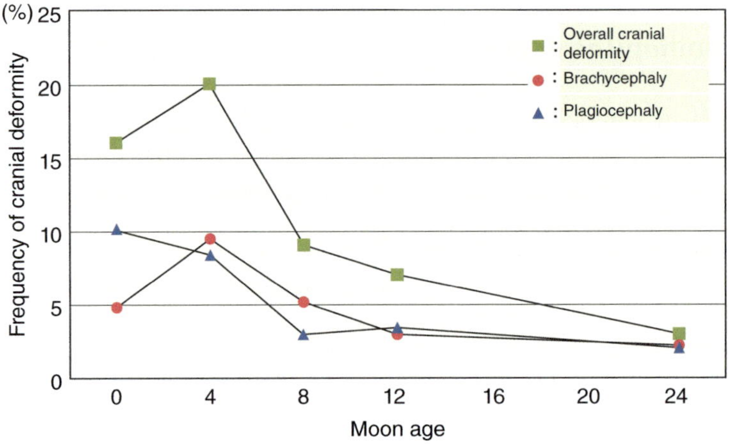

Fig. 1.1 Trends in incidence of cranial deformity by age (created from Reference [5]. Newborns born in a single New Zealand hospital in 2001 were followed up to 2 years of age. Two hundred children were enrolled in this cohort study, and 181 were observed for the presence or absence of cranial deformity by age 2 years. The incidence of cranial deformity was highest at 4 months of age, approximately 20%. Although cranial deformity was noted, many were followed up without intervention, and only nine cases underwent repositioning interventions. At 2 years of age, six (3.3%) had a residual cranial deformity. (©Nabeco)

deformity tends to improve after infants gain head control but persists in some individuals. That is, the position of the head during sleep is once fixed with deviation, the deformation itself progresses further, and finally, the cranial deformation becomes permanent as the skull bone fusion is completed.

2 Types and Mechanisms

Cranial deformities are classified into plagiocephaly, brachycephaly, and dolichocephaly according to the types, with plagiocephaly being the most common. Conversely, cranial deformities that occur due to premature synostosis of cranial sutures are the result of congenital abnormalities and should be considered completely separate from positional cranial deformities.

Causes of cranial deformity can be broadly divided into prenatal and postnatal causes (Table 1.2). However, the influence of postnatal causes is quite strong. Prenatal factors include physical pressure on the head due to abnormal fetal presentation, such as breech or lateral position, and persistent external pressure from other infants in multiple pregnancy. In addition, uterine abnormalities also play a role. Cranial deformity may already exist at birth due to intrauterine pressure. Once the head position is fixed after birth due to the prenatal deformation, there is a possibility that the cranial deformation will progress further. Similarly, there are several postnatal factors including preterm infants, developmental disorders, first child, male infants, muscular torticollis, treatment for hip dislocation, and cerebral palsy [1, 6, 7]. Infants with movement disorders, muscular torticollis, and hip joint dislocation are often treated for plagiocephaly and brachycephaly because they cannot move their heads freely.

Because preterm infants needs to spend long duration in the neonatal intensive care unit (NICU), and they are usually managed in the prone position with their faces turned to the side for a long time, cranial deformity and dolichocephaly are common. Even in term infants, plagiocephaly occurs due to a condition called the habit of facing, asymmetrical head turn preference. Conversely, sleeping on the back with the head always facing upward causes brachycephaly. Therefore, it has been reported that the frequency of positional cranial deformity can be reduced simply by adjusting the head position during sleep [8].

Table 1.2 Risk factors for positional cranial deformity (created from References [1, 6, 7])

Prenatal	After birth
• Abnormal fetal position such as breech or lateral position	• Supine sleep
• Multiple pregnancy	• Preterm infants
• Uterine malformation	• Small-for-date infants
	• First child
	• Male sex
	• Muscular torticollis
	• Treatment for hip dislocation
	• Cerebral palsy

3 Effects on Development

3.1 Reported by a Systematic Review

Conventionally, positional cranial deformity has been regarded as a cosmetic concern in adults, and its pathological significance has been questioned. However, there is a possibility that skull deformity may develop into facial bone deformation, and there are cases where it cannot be ignored as a mere cosmetic problem [9]. Furthermore, many reports have suggested that cranial deformity may negatively impact motor development in infants, and finally, systematic reviews have strongly suggested its association with impaired neuromotor development [10].

Martiniuk et al. retrieved 1315 papers on the relationship between cranial deformity and neuromotor development that were published up to 2016. From these, 35 papers were extracted as scientific studies on the relationship between cranial deformity and developmental disorders, and 19 with strong scientific grounds were finally analyzed. Table 1.3 shows the number of papers that recognized the relationship between cranial deformity and impairment of neuromotor development by developmental tests. Overall, 13 of the 19 publications showed positional cranial deformity and impaired neuromotor development. Furthermore, among these reports, when only five papers whose analysis method was scientifically judged to be accurate were analyzed, again four reports showed a significant relationship with neurodevelopmental disorders. Therefore, positional cranial deformities are likely to be a risk factor for neuromotor developmental disorders in children. However, most of the reports are on development up to 2 years of age, and the intellectual development later on is not completely studied.

Wallace et al. followed up 235 children with cranial deformity until school age (mean age 9 years) and measured intelligence quotient (IQ) and reported that there was no significant correlation between cranial deformity and IQ [11]. Therefore, impairment of neuromotor development in infancy due to cranial deformity cannot be judged as a permanent impairment.

Table 1.3 Relationship between cranial deformity and neuromotor development (systematic review) (created from reference [10])

Developmental testing method	Number of papers considered[a]	Relationship with developmental disorders Number of papers[a]
Objective developmental test[b]	11	9
Questionnaire-type developmental test[c]	10	3
Physiological test[d]	3	2

[a] Papers using multiple testing methods were taught in duplicate
[b] Developmental tests conducted by examiners such as the Bayley scale
[c] Developmental testing using questionnaires such as Ages & Stages Questionnaires (ASQ-3)
[d] Judgment using electrophysiological tests such as auditory brainstem response

3.2 Reports of Preterm Infants

Conversely, preterm infants have a higher frequency of cranial deformity than full-term infants, and it is said that cranial deformity strongly affects neuromotor development in infants [12]. Preterm infants are often managed in the prone position in the NICU for a long time, which results in a vertically elongated and horizontally flattened head. Posture also becomes left–right asymmetrical, and as a result, the range of spontaneous movement is restricted [13]. Therefore, cranial deformity in premature infants may lead to deformities in the infant's general posture, and such movement restriction is likely to negatively impact the infant's future neuromotor development [14]. Cranial deformity is a systemic problem for preterm infants and is a serious problem that affects future development. However, it has been reported that early intervention improves developmental delay due to cranial deformity in preterm infants [15]. In other words, in preterm infants who are at high risk for delayed neuromotor development, it is important to consider the impact of cranial deformity on the future neuromotor development of the infant and implement early intervention if necessary.

From the above, positional cranial deformity cannot be regarded as a mere transient problem in infancy or a cosmetic problem. Given the persistent problems beyond infancy, the negative impact on neuromotor development, and the increased risk in preterm infants, positional cranial deformity should be considered a pathologic condition requiring intervention according to the severity of deformity.

Although intervention might be introduced for positional cranial deformity including improving sleep posture with pillows and orthotic treatment with helmets, it is more important to establish a system for accurate diagnosis and early prevention and intervention for cranial deformity in infancy.

References

1. Ballardini E, Sisti M, Basaglia N, et al. Prevalence and characteristics of positional plagiocephaly in healthy full-term infants at 8-12 weeks of life. Eur J Pediatr. 2018;177:1547–54.
2. Mawji A, Vollman AR, Hatifield J, et al. The incidence of positional plagiocephaly: a cohort study. Pediatrics. 2013;132:298–304.
3. American Academy of Pediatrics AAP task force on infant positioning and SIDS. Positioning and SIDS. Pediatrics. 1992;89:1120–6.
4. Kane AA, Mitchell LE, Craven KP, et al. Observations on a recent increase in plagiocephaly without synostosis. Pediatrics. 1996;97:877–85.
5. Hutchison BL, Hutchison LAD, Thompson JMD, et al. Plagiocephaly and Brachycephaly in the first two years of life: a prospective cohort study. Pediatrics. 2008;114:970–80.
6. McKinney CM, Cunningham ML, Holtet V, et al. A case-control study of infant, maternal and perinatal characteristics associated with deformational plagiocephaly. Paediatr Perinat Epidemiol. 2009;23:332–45.
7. Mawji A, Vollman AR, Fung T, et al. Risk factors for positional plagiocephaly and appropriate time frames for preventing messaging. Pediatr Child Health. 2014;19:423–7.

8. Cavalier A, Picot MC, Artiaga C, et al. Prevention of deformational plagiocephaly in neonates. Early Hum Dev. 2011;87:537–43.
9. Yu CC, Wong FH, Lo LJ, et al. Craniofacial deformity in patients with uncorrected congenital muscular torticollis: an assessment from three-dimensional computed tomography imaging. Plast Reconstr Surg. 2004;113:24–33.
10. Martiniuk ALC, Vujovich-Dunn C, Park M, et al. Plagiocephaly and developmental delay: a systematic review. J Dev Behav Pediatr. 2017;38:67–78.
11. Wallace ER, Ola C, Leroux BG, et al. Prediction of school-age IQ, academic achievement, and motor skills in children with positional plagiocephaly. Paediatr Child Health. 2021;26:e132–7.
12. Nuysink J, MJC E, van Haastert IC, et al. Clinical course of asymmetric motor performance and deformational plagiocephaly in very preterm infants. J Pediatr. 2013;263:658–65.
13. Nuysink J, Eijsermans MJC, van Haastert IC, et al. Prevalence and predictors of idiopathic asymmetry in infants born preterm. Early Hum Dev. 2012;88:387–92.
14. Uchio Y, Hasegawa M, Ikai T, et al. Comparison of upper extremity activity in very low birth weight infants and full-term infants at corrected 1 month. Phys Ther. 2018;45:347–57.
15. Uchio Y, Shima N, Nakamura K, et al. Effects of continued positioning pillow use until a corrected age of six months on cranial deformation and neurodevelopment in preterm infants: a prospective case-control study. Early Hum Dev. 2020;148:105137.

Part II
Assessment and Evaluation of Positional Plagiocephaly at Grouped Infant Checkups or Private Pediatric Clinics

Chapter 2
Response to Cranial Deformities on the Day of Infant Health Checkup and in a Maternity Ward (Hospital)

Isao Kusakawa

1 Cranial Deformity Progression and Diagnosis

Here, we explain how the deformation of the infant's head begins and how it progresses over time. Based on the child's growth and development, it is important to take appropriate, reasonable, and safe measures at an appropriate time.

1.1 Maternal–Fetal Period

As delivery approaches, the baby's head is usually the leading part and enters the mother's pelvic cavity. Rotating the body toward the narrow birth canal, the child is finally born into this world.

There are three ways to express the position of the fetus in the uterus: "fetal presentation," "fetal orientation," and "fetal posture," each of which refers to the posture shown in Fig. 2.1.

At the end of pregnancy, the fetus turns in preparation for delivery. In a normal state, it is facing the back side of the mother's body (backward facing). The face and body are slightly tilted to the left or right (first or second fetal position), with the neck bent forward and head down (cephalic position). It is said that the first and second fetal orientations are normal, but the first is said to be more prevalent [1–3].

When the head of the fetus gets fixed in the birth canal, the fetus is often born with a deformation of the head due to pressure; these deformations often result in left–right asymmetries. Because babies pass through a narrow birth canal during

I. Kusakawa (✉)
Baby's Head Reshaping Clinic, Tokyo, Japan
e-mail: kusakawa.isao@baby-helmet.com

S. Kusuda et al. (eds.), *Handbook of Positional Plagiocephaly*,
https://doi.org/10.1007/978-981-97-9164-4_2

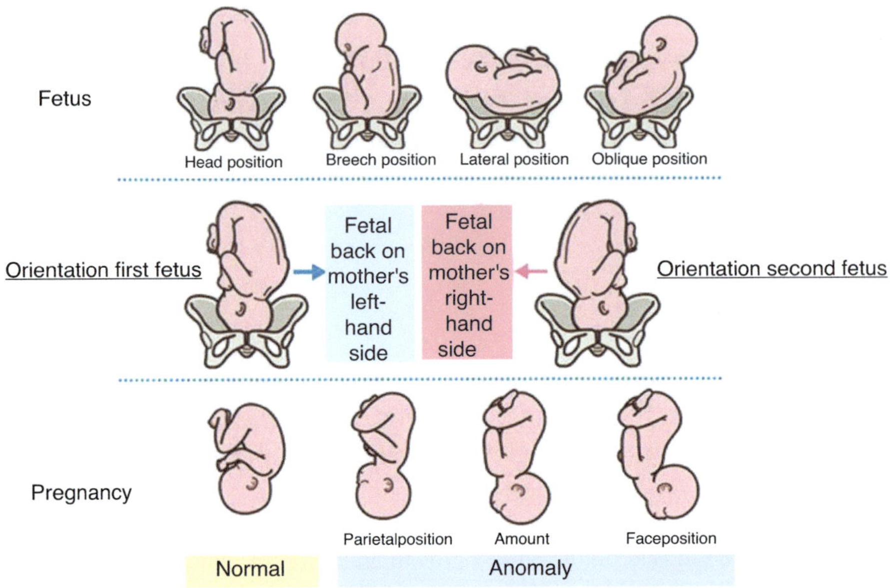

Fig. 2.1 The posture of the fetus inside the mother's body (from nursing room! illustration collection). (©Nabeco)

delivery, they may be born with their skull bones overlapping each other, which is called bone polymerization.

Point: A baby's head is very soft, and the effects of delivery are inevitable.

1.2 During Hospitalization after Birth

Most hospitalized infants are placed in baby beds known as cots (Fig. 2.2). A baby in a cot is laid on a baby mattress with sheets, towels, and so on. The first thing that health-care workers who care for newborns need to be aware of is to check for distortions in the shape of the head due to the position in the womb or the effects of delivery. If there is any deformation in the head (horizontal deviation, partial flattening, bone polymerization, etc.), it is important to gently move the head so that it does not remain in the same position so as to avoid aggravating the deformation.

Cephalohematoma should not be overlooked during hospitalization. Cephalohematoma is bleeding under the periosteum of the skull due to an external force applied to the head when passing through a narrow birth canal during delivery. Because the bleeding is under the periosteum, it does not cross the bony suture line. In many cases, the diagnosis cannot be made immediately after birth, and the diagnosis becomes definite from around the third day after birth when the hematoma becomes conspicuous. Cephalohematoma usually does not require any special

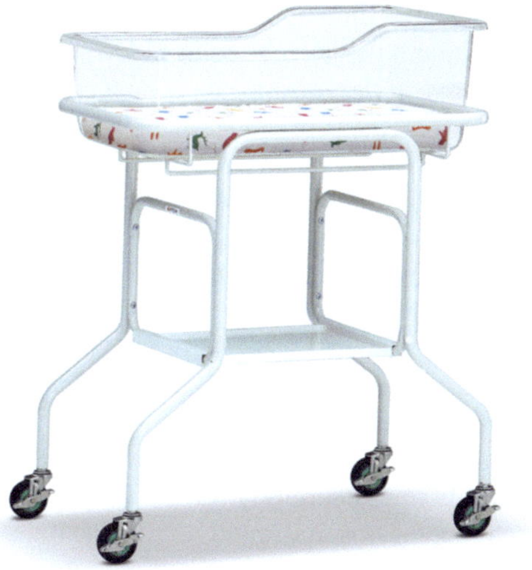

Fig. 2.2 Baby cot An example of what is often used as a medical crib in delivery facilities, perinatal centers, and so on. The mattress is usually used with a sheet, towel, and so on (Photo courtesy of Atom Medical). (©Nabeco)

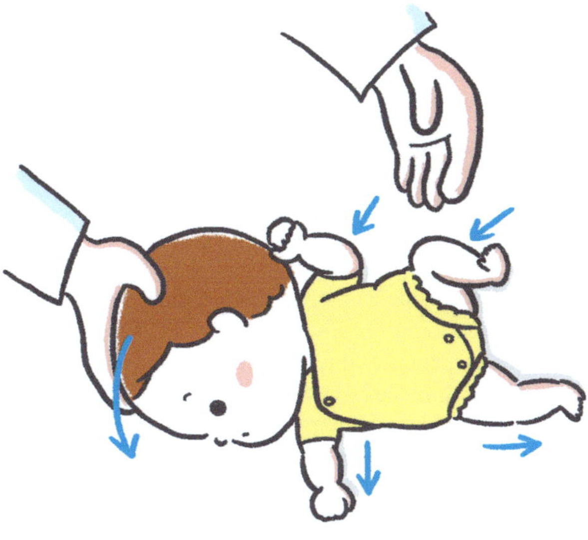

Fig. 2.3 Asymmetric tonic neck reflex fencing style. (©Nabeco)

treatment and can be cured in a few weeks to half a year just by follow-up. The positional cranial deformity is likely to occur due to laterality, and care must be taken when dealing with it.

When moving the direction of the baby's head during this period, it is useful to know the baby's natural posture. The natural leg position is that which is easy for the baby to take naturally and is related to the orientation of the head. Primitive reflexes are often involved in this limb position, and the asymmetrical tonic neck reflex is related to the direction of the head. As shown in Fig. 2.3, when the head is turned to the left without moving the body, the left upper and lower limbs are extended, and the right upper and lower limbs are flexed (fencing style). Conversely, this means that if the head is facing sideways, the position of the hand is determined. This primitive reflex disappears 5–6 months after birth, and rolling over begins around this time [4].

Knowing that the position of the hands will naturally change when there is a change in the position of a baby's head, the baby can be made to adopt a posture that he or she will not object to (natural leg position).

In any case, what is important at this stage is to change the child's posture so that gravity does not apply to only one part of the head. In addition, cuddling is also an important way to free the head from the pressure of gravity.

Point: Check for cranial deformities related to delivery early after birth and take appropriate measures.

[Explanation to family] Babies pass through a narrow birth canal when they are born, so it is not uncommon for the shape of the head to differ from side to side. After leaving the hospital, gently turn the baby's head to avoid the baby always turning in the same direction. When bathing, observe the shape of your baby's head and make sure there are no flat areas on it. If any such areas are observed, try to make sure that part isn't placed against the bed when your baby is laid down to rest or sleep.

1.3 The Neonatal Period Until the 1-Month Checkup After Discharge

Babies discharged from the hospital 4–5 days to 1 week after birth begin their daily lives at home using a crib, a bed-in-bed, a baby comforter (bedding futon (Japanese style)), or bedding for adults. Often, the baby sleeps on these beddings (not limited to sleep time, but the time the baby is laid). This time constitutes almost all the time outside any time the baby is being held for breastfeeding, crying, bathing time, and diaper changing time. Normally, breastfeeding takes approximately 30 minutes at a time, 8–12 times a day. It takes approximately 10–15 min for exhaustion after breastfeeding. Bathing should be done for 30 min at most, changing diapers for about 5 min, 10–12 times a day, and holding and cradling the child indoors for about 15 min, 7–8 times a day. After subtracting these hours from the 24 h, the infant will be lying on the bed for 11–12 h.

Infants at this age tend to move their heads less on their own while lying down, especially when part of the skull is flattened and "sitting well" relative to the plane of the bed. Even if they try to move their head, they cannot properly move it; hence, they tend to assume the same posture. During this period, instead of leaving the child lying down just because he or she sleeps excessively, it is important to be conscious, hold the child in arms, or change the direction of the head to release the pressure of gravity from the same part of the head.

Point: Do not let the baby lie down in the same position, but turn its head consciously.

1.4 1-Month Checkup

Since the 1-month checkup is often the first opportunity for the neonate to be examined after discharge from the Obstetrics ward, it is important to confirm perinatal risk factors, such as vitality, respiratory and feeding status, weight gain, and muscle tone. The focus is on the examination and evaluation of neurologic abnormalities in patients. Table 2.1 shows the examination findings of the 1-month-old health checkup in the "Infants Health Checkup Physical Examination Manual" published in March 2018 [5, 6]. Although there are descriptions of congenital malformations, neither pathologic cranial deformities (premature cranial suture synostosis) nor clinical findings related to positional cranial deformities are unfortunately described.

Growth is confirmed by referring to the growth curve published in the Maternal and Child Health Handbook, but height measurement during this period is often inaccurate, and evidently, weight is the most important indicator. However, at this time, please also pay attention to the head circumference growth curve. The head circumference is just the length around the skull and does not represent the shape of the skull. However, we must know that the head circumference increases by approximately 3 cm in 1 month and the slope of the growth curve is steep. This rapid growth of the head circumference means the growth of the brain, and this growth

Table 2.1 Examination findings of 1-month-old health checkup positions

1. Physical developmental abnormalities
2. Psychiatric disorders: Eyes do not meet, does not respond to sounds or voices
3. Convulsions
4. Abnormalities in motor development: Abnormalities in posture/abnormality in locomotor activity
5. Nervous system abnormalities: Muscle tone abnormalities, reflex abnormalities
6. Sensory abnormalities: Visual abnormalities, auditory abnormalities
7. Blood disorders: Anemia, others
8. Skin diseases: Eczema, others
9. Hip joint: Limited opening and excretion, not M-shaped leg opening
10. Torticollis
11. Cardiovascular disease: Heart murmur, others
12. Respiratory disease
13. Gastrointestinal disease: Abdominal bloating/abdominal mass, inguinal hernia, umbilical hernia, constipation, and so on
14. Genitourinary disorders: Undescended testicles, external genital abnormalities, and so on
15. Inborn error of metabolism
16. Congenital malformation (head, face, limbs, trunk, etc.)
17. Other abnormalities (such as child abuse)

pushes up the skull from the inside, that is, the growth of bilateral symmetry. As an example, the head circumference growth curve of a boy is shown in Fig. 2.4 [7].

The growth of the head circumference is the steepest until about 3 months after birth, and thereafter the slope of the head circumference growth curve gradually becomes gentle, and the skull also changes around 9–10 months when the infant stands up on its own and gradually becomes stronger.

Among the examination findings of the 1-month-old health checkup, there are items to check for the presence or absence of torticollis and check for the presence or absence of restriction on excretion (congenital hip dislocation). There is also a report pointing out the relationship between the two, which may result in positional cranial deformity. Therefore, if both are recognized, it is necessary to confirm the presence or absence of cranial deformity more carefully [8].

When the cranial deformity is observed, check by palpation whether there is a bulge of the bone along the cranial suture line (one of the signs to positively suspect cranial suture early synostosis).

Point: In the 1-month checkup, check for flattening of any part of the head (the result of gravity being applied to the same place). If deformity is observed and there is no bulging bone along the cranial suture line (a finding that positively suggests early cranial suture synostosis), the patient should first be instructed not to continue applying gravity to the same part of the head daily.

[Explanation to family members] When observing the head and finding a flat part on the skull, it is better not to ask the parents about the shape of the skull, such as "Does the baby tend to turn to one side?" It is easier for them to understand if you start by asking about the baby's so-called orientation preference: (1) "Why did you notice that?" → (2) "Because it is flat?" → (3) "Does the baby's orientation

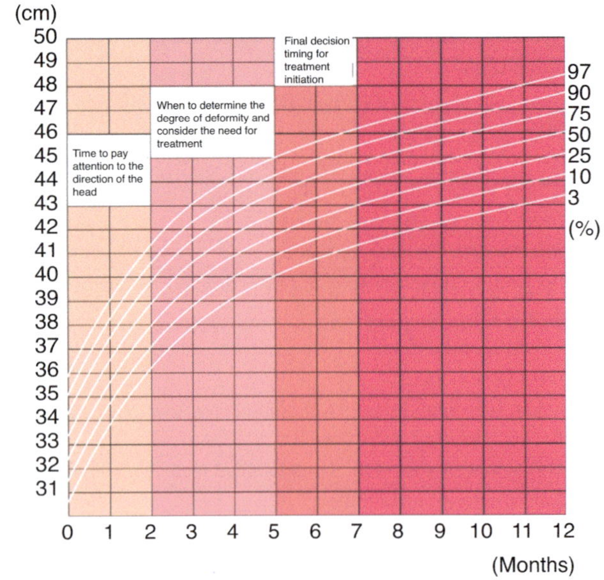

Fig. 2.4 Growth curve of the head circumference for infants (boys) (2000 survey)The evaluation of the degree of positional cranial deformity and the guideline for the start of treatment are presented. (©Nabeco)

preference create a flat part?" Therefore, the reason why it becomes flat will be explained.

Guide them as follows: specifically, the baby's head is heavy, and at this stage, the baby cannot move the head freely by itself. Therefore, in the future, I advise you to avoid as much as possible the posture where gravity is applied to this flat part. Regarding the use of donut pillows (Fig. 2.5), which are frequently asked about, it is not recommended at this stage because the neck bends forward and is dangerous (Fig. 2.6).

1.5 Between the 1-Month Health Checkup and the 3–4-Month Health Checkup

This is the most critical period for positional cranial deformity. Especially for 1–2 months, the skull is still tender. Moreover, it is not yet the age when the child can move his or her head freely and skillfully. Therefore, when gravity is applied to a part of the skull and causes deformation (appearance of a flat part), it is possible to frequently passively move the direction of the head so that gravity is applied evenly to other areas.

Conversely, considering the sleeping conditions of infants, after 1 month, they begin to establish a feeding rhythm and gradually come to sleep for a long period. During sleep, if the cranium has a partially flat portion because of deformation due to gravity, the infant often sleeps with that comfortable portion facing down. This results in increased deformity, which unfortunately is not good for cranial deformity.

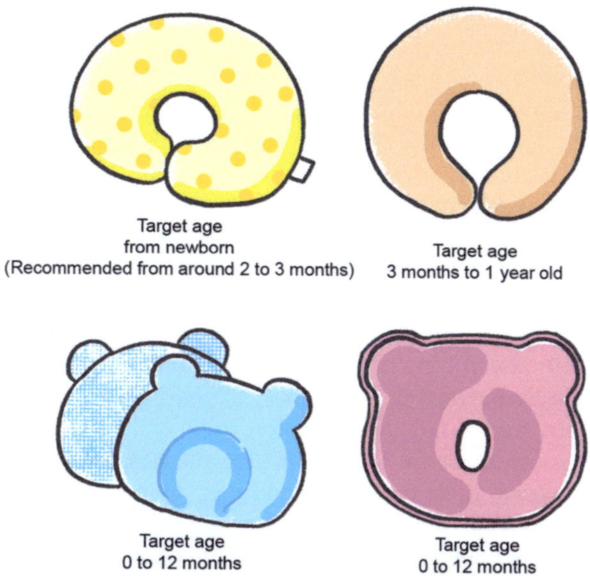

Fig. 2.5 Various shapes of donut pillows. There are various types, but basically, most of them are suitable for 2 to 3 months old. Those suitable for newborns are U-shaped, not O-shaped donuts. (©Nabeco)

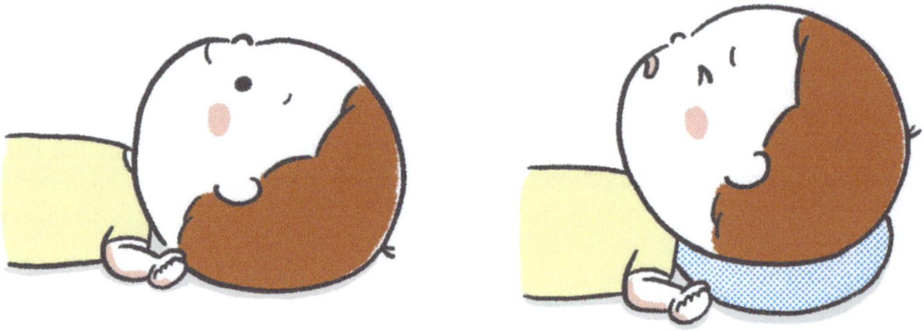

Fig. 2.6 Risk of airway obstruction with donut pillows. Risk of airway obstruction as the neck is flexed and the lower jaw is pressed against the chest. (©Nabeco)

Families who dreamed of a baby who would sleep soundly would naturally think, "Since I've been able to sleep for a long time, I want to let him sleep quietly." From the perspective of deformation, caution is required, such as gently turning the head during sleep.

Point: It is important to adopt a posture that does not continuously apply gravity to the flat part of the skull that has been created.

1.6 3–4-Month-Old Health Checkup

The 3–4-month-old health checkup is the time to get rid of primitive reflexes such as the Moro reflex. This is the stage when the baby acquires functions such as sitting on the neck (fixed neck), coordinated hand movements, and tracking, and many facial expressions such as comforting and smiling. Although there are descriptions of congenital malformations here as well, examination findings related to cranial deformities are unfortunately not described, with the exceptions of torticollis and hip developmental dysplasia of the hip joints.

Therefore, we describe in detail the follow-up related to cranial deformation, other than general medical examination items.

Babies that have grown repeatedly through breastfeeding and sleep become able to move their heads and follow moving objects freely at this age. The fixed neck progresses, and the control of head movement improves.

However, as cranial deformation progresses, this movement of the head is often restricted. If there is a clear left–right difference when checking the tracking situation by moving an object that the child is interested in, it is often due to cranial deformation. If there is no deformation or the degree of deformation is slight, tracking can be performed by moving the head smoothly and nearly symmetrically. However, if the cranial deformity is strong and the orientation is strong, the head does not move in a direction that is not usually seen. The baby follows with just their eyes. In addition, even if a child who can follow up by moving the head direction without any difference at this point has cranial deformation, the deformation is likely not progressing. It is thought that it may be a period in the middle of natural remission. In any case, it is important to observe the presence or absence of cranial deformity during this period as well, and particularly, if left–right differences are observed during follow-up search, it is necessary to carefully evaluate the severity of the condition. Figure 2.7 shows the lateral difference in tracking.

At this stage, infants usually move their heads freely without left–right differences. In addition, as the body stabilizes and stays awake longer, the time spent sitting on a bouncer or baby rack (Fig. 2.8) increases, as well as on the bed. As a result, the chances of gravity concentrating on the same part of the skull gradually decrease, and the deformity becomes less noticeable with growth. Contrarily, more than half of the children will sleep continuously for about 6 hours at night at this time. During this period, children who can move their heads freely can change their head position even during sleep, but when children who have a strong orientation tendency fall asleep, they cannot move their heads on their own but can sit comfortably. They spend ample time in the position. Therefore, there are many cases where the deformation due to growth does not progress. This is the time to determine the

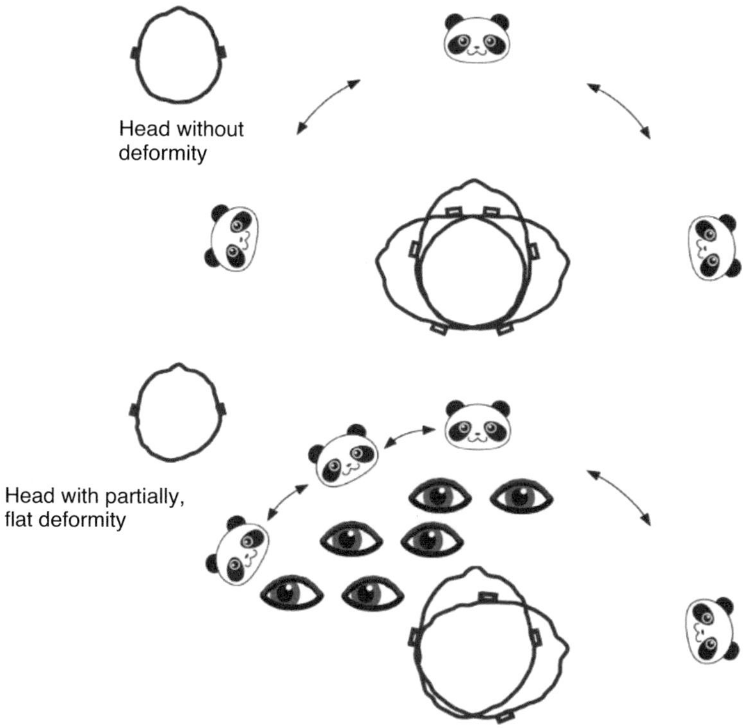

Fig. 2.7 Tracking. Top: No deformation (move the head to see the object)Bottom: When there is cranial deformity/orientation (try to look at the nonflat side by moving only the eyeballs without moving the head). (©Nabeco)

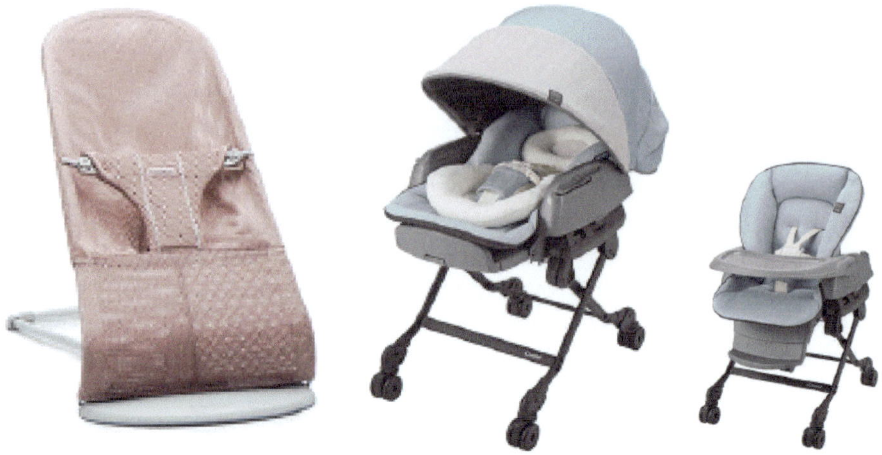

Fig. 2.8 Example of a bouncer (left) and baby rack (right). Left: Many bouncers have a net-like back made of cloth or something similar, and instead of supporting a part of the skull on a flat surface, they support the skull as if it is wrapped around it (photo courtesy of Baby Bjorn). Right: The baby rack can be adjusted in height, and some have functions such as automatic rocking (photo courtesy of Combi). (©Nabeco)

need for aggressive intervention for cranial deformities (mainly plagiocephaly). The criteria for judging severity are as follows:

1. Obvious left–right difference in pursuit and inability to turn one's face to the opposite side of the flattened skull.
2. Flattened cranial ear deviated forward.
3. Flattened cranial forehead slightly protruding and so on.

In addition to plagiocephaly mentioned earlier, other cranial deformities include dolichocephaly, in which the head is lengthened in the anteroposterior diameter, and brachycephaly, which shortens the anteroposterior diameter. At that time, if there is a clear influence on movements such as tracking, consider the same.

Points: Around 3–4 months of age is the time to consider the severity of cranial deformity and refer to a specialized medical institution.

[Explanation to the family] While observing the follow-up together with the family of the child who has a left–right difference in the follow-up test and confirming that there is a left–right difference, I said, "Your child is moving with a left-right difference." As I lift the baby's head and observe the deformed part, I explain, "It may be difficult for the baby to heal on its own because it cannot move on its own."'In addition, if there is a positional displacement of the ear, protrusion of the forehead, and so on, explain to them and proceed with the introduction and discussion to a specialized medical institution. At this time, it should be added that there is a bulge on the cranial suture line (possible premature union), or even if there is no bulge, there is a disease called premature cranial suture synostosis.

In addition, at this time, since helmet correction treatment for positional cranial deformity is costly, we started by introducing it as one of the options, and the family members felt guilty that they could not receive treatment for financial reasons. However, if the family wants treatment from the beginning, early consultation should be considered to prevent delaying the start of treatment.

1.7 After 3–4 Months Health Checkup

Recently, as awareness of cranial deformity has increased, cases of parents worrying about cranial deformity are increasing after 5–6 months after the 3–4-month health checkup. However, as mentioned in the head circumference growth curve, if possible, the cranial deformity should be treated with neck fixation, and at 3–4 months after the start of follow-up, it is possible to evaluate whether treatment is indicated at a specialized medical institution and start helmet correction treatment. It is the most effective treatment, and the longer it is delayed, the less effective it will be. Many specialized medical institutions start treatment for infants up to 6 months old because the effect is not zero, although the effect is reduced. However, even if a cranial deformity is found at the checkup for a 6–7-month-old child, if a developmental milestone such as rolling over is normal, and if the family does not seem to be concerned about it, we believe it is appropriate to end the medical checkup without mentioning this matter.

References

1. Susumu J. That is why there are many fetuses of the first head position, first classification. Midwifery Magazine. 2013;67(10):869–71.
2. Mitani S. On the statistics of postpartum positions. Deliv Anesth. 1966;16:134–5.
3. Morooka M, et al. Fetal rotation (assessment of normal/abnormal rotation). Perinatal Care. 2013;32(5):435–43.
4. Kono H, editor. Bedside newborn examination, vol. 2009. 2nd ed. Tokyo: Nanzando; 2009. p. 119.
5. 2017 Child/Child-rearing Support Promotion Research Project, Research on the preparation of "Health Guidance Manual (provisional name)" and "Physical Examination Manual (provisional name)" for infant health checkups, "Infants Health Checkup Physical Examination Manual" National Research and Development Agency National Center for Child Health and Development March 2018.
6. 2018–2020 Health, Labor and Welfare Scientific Research Subsidy (Comprehensive Research Project for Next-Generation Nurturing Overcoming Childhood Diseases) Breaks to promote the development of physically, mentally, and socially healthy children A study for the provision of health and medical care systems that do not require care, "Revised infant health examination physical examination manual" (in Japanese).
7. 2011 Health, Labor and Welfare Science Research Grant (Basic research project for nurturing the next generation, such as overcoming childhood diseases) "Statistical analysis of infant

physical development survey and research on its method and utilization" Infant physical development evaluation manual, p. 28.
8. Asagai Y. Other diseases that should be noted in health checkups: orthopedic surgery. Pediatrics. 2021;53(3):395–7.

Chapter 3
Intervention for Skull Deformity and Referral to Specialized Medical Institutions

Shigeharu Hosono

1 Ingenuity in the Position and Direction of Laying Down [1]

In many homes, the crib is usually placed with one long side against the wall and the other side with a living space. After returning home from the obstetric ward, the infant is placed on the bed with alternating head-side and foot-side positions after each feeding. Since the infant faces the direction of interest (toward the living space), it is no longer necessary to always sleep in the same direction.

For children with plagiocephaly and a clear preference for a particular face direction, take the time to deliberately change the face direction to the position opposite of preference. Specifically, first, the orientation of the infant's face during sleep is observed. If there is a clear right- or left-facing tendency in the child's face orientation, the parent should position the child on the opposite side of the child's preferred sleeping direction when awake or place an object of interest next to the child (Fig. 3.1).

S. Hosono (✉)
Saitama Medical Center, Jichi Medical University, Saitama, Japan
e-mail: hosono.s@jichi.ac.jp

S. Kusuda et al. (eds.), *Handbook of Positional Plagiocephaly*,
https://doi.org/10.1007/978-981-97-9164-4_3

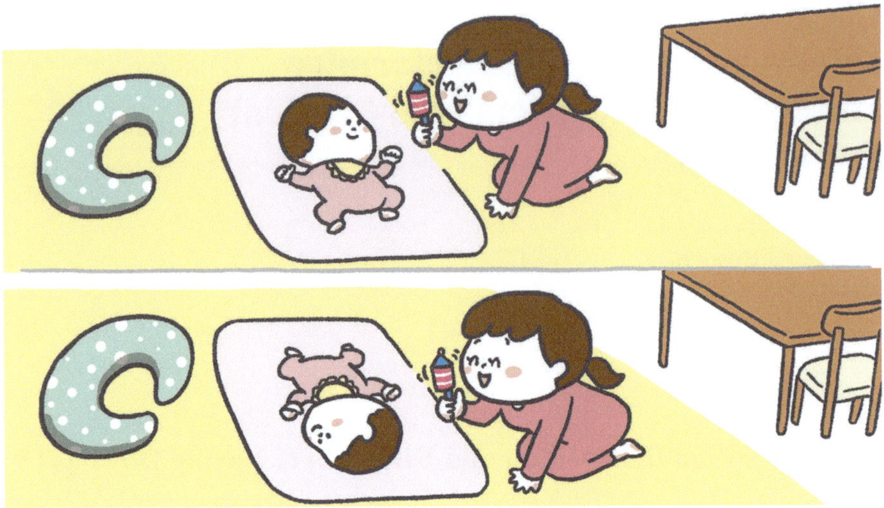

Fig. 3.1 Adjusting the direction the child wants to face. (©Nabeco)

2 Introduction of Tummy Time

2.1 What Is Tummy Time?

Tummy time is not defined in the Japanese Association of Medical Sciences Medical Terminology Dictionary web. In general, the terms "prone practice (play)" and "tummy practice (play)" are used as a method to encourage the acquisition of a fixed head. This consists of making time for the child to lie face down under the supervision of a guardian or the like when the child is awake.

Until the baby can roll over, if it lies on its stomach and sinks into the mattress with its face facing the midline, it will not be able to shift its face position, and its mouth and nose will be blocked by the mattress, causing suffocation (Fig. 3.2).

The "AAP Committee on Practice and Ambulatory Medicine and Section on Neurologic Surgery" by the American Academy of Pediatrics recommends that the tummy time be implemented for a certain period to prevent flattening of the occiput and improve the development of the upper shoulder girdle [2].

2.2 When to Start

The AAP recommends that once a newborn has returned home from a delivery facility, the tummy time should be started 2–3 times a day for 3–5 min, immediately after the baby wakes up after changing diapers [3]. If the child is willing to do it, gradually extend it to at least 30–60 min in the prone position [4]. This should be carried out consciously during the period until the baby can crawl on its stomach or all fours.

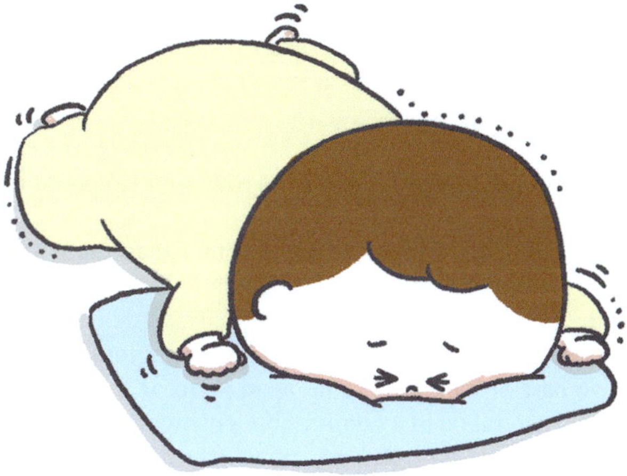

Fig. 3.2 Dangerous lying on the stomach. If a child lies face down on soft bedding when it cannot move its face, its nose and mouth will be buried in the bedding and cause suffocation. (©Nabeco)

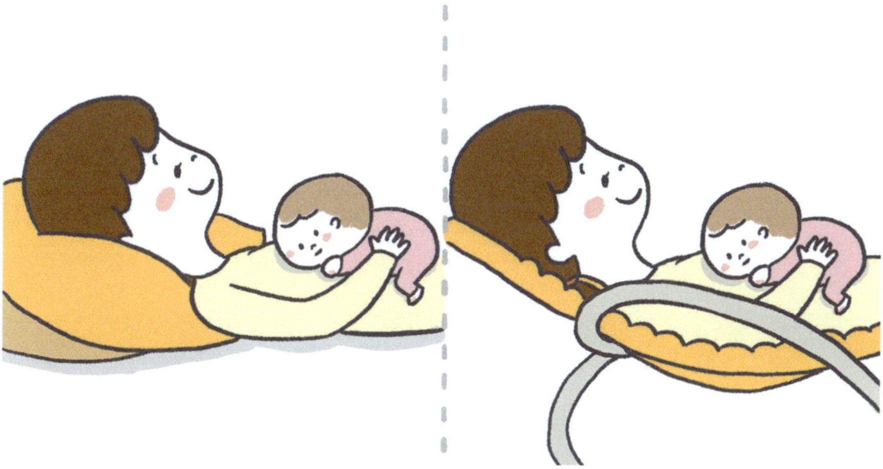

Fig. 3.3 Lying down on the chest. (©Nabeco)

2.3 Methods

Depending on the child's developmental status and preferences, try the following strategies.

2.3.1 Lying Face Down on parent's Chest (Fig. 3.3)

During periods when the head cannot be lifted, the baby can be held prone on the parent's chest. There is no need to remove clothes and apply direct skin-to-skin contact, as in mother–infant early contact and kangaroo care, and it is possible to perform the treatment with the clothes on. In the case of mothers, make sure that the mouth and nose are not blocked by the breasts. Parents can relax in a rocking chair, even if they are not necessarily lying on bedding.

2.3.2 The Parent Lays on the Side and Looks at the child's Face (Fig. 3.4)

When the head cannot be lifted, other than the above method [1], the mother or father should lie on the side of the child and look in the direction the child is facing. If the baby does not have plagiocephaly, do this with alternating facial turns throughout the day. If plagiocephaly is a problem, turn the face to the side so that the concave part of the back of the head is up. If the child can see the parent's face, the parent should be in a comfortable position.

2.3.3 Child and Parent Lie Face Down on the Same Axis (Fig. 3.5)

If the infant can lift its head briefly, the infant and parent lie prone on the same axis. If the parent's face is at a high position from the floor, the child will find it difficult to make eye contact, and the child will dislike it. If head lift strength is weak, start with short durations and combine with other techniques. If the baby can lift its head longer, do this method alone.

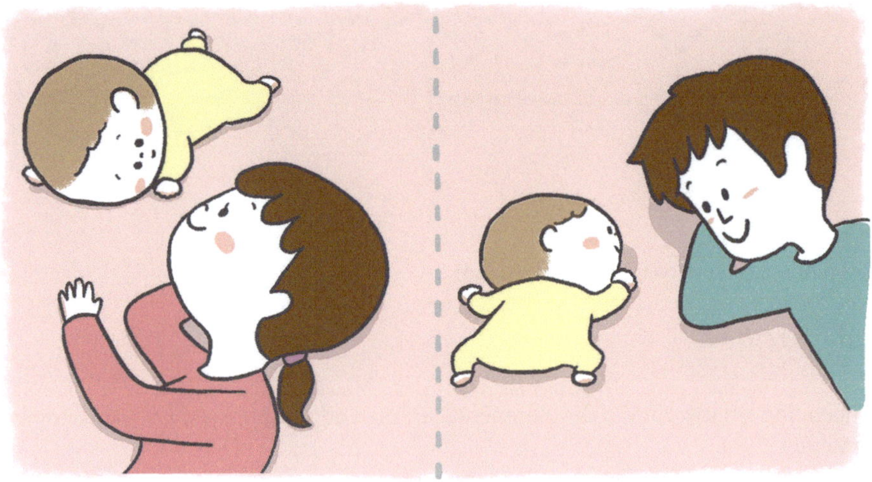

Fig. 3.4 Parents lying on their sides and looking at the child's face. (©Nabeco)

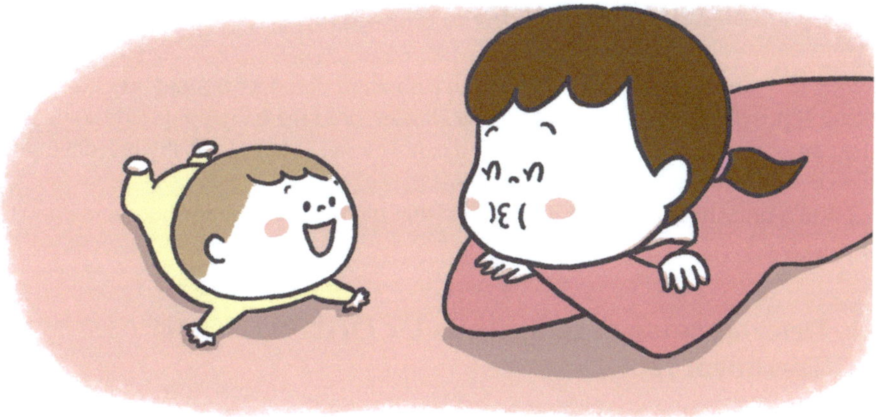

Fig. 3.5 Child and parent lie face down on the same axis. (©Nabeco)

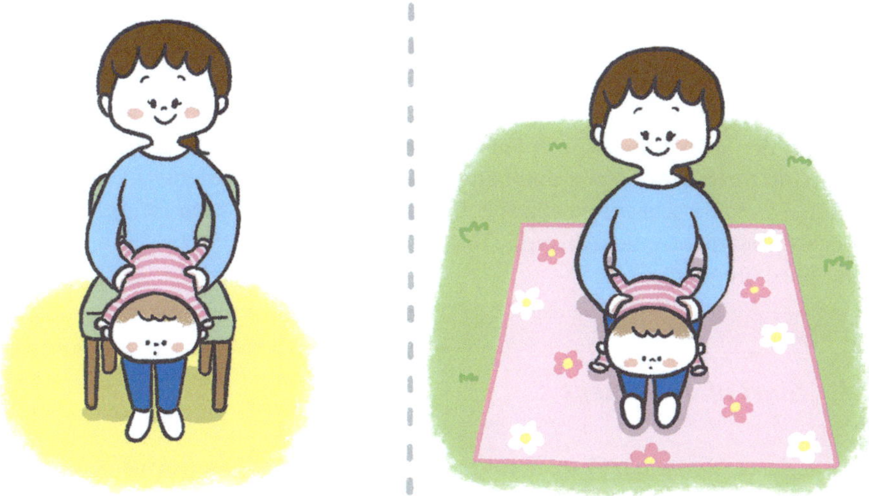

Fig. 3.6 How to lie face down on the thigh. (©Nabeco)

2.3.4 Lay Face Down on thigh [4] (Fig. 3.6)

Place the child face down on the thigh in a seated position where the parent either sits on a chair or puts the feet on the floor. Support the child's head so that it is in line with the body. The advantage is that it can be done outdoors, but care must be taken because the infant's face cannot be observed, and it may be difficult to balance the position of the femur and the infant if one is not used to it. Raise and lower both feet slowly and swing slowly from side to side to provide stimulation.

3 Ingenuity in Daily Life [5]

When the baby is awake, try to keep it in a position that does not put pressure on the head. If possible, rather than laying in a stroller, hold the baby on its side so that the flat part of the head is not down, or use a carrier strap to hold the baby in front before the neck is stabilized.

When breastfeeding, hold the baby so that the flat head side is not facing down.

4 Determination of Indications for Orthotic Helmet Treatment [2]

Mild plagiocephaly, which progresses to moderate despite the introduction of prevention and treatment by positioning as described above, and facial asymmetry caused by severe plagiocephaly are no longer believed to spontaneously resolve. The only cure is orthotic helmet treatment. The principle of this treatment is to use helmet orthosis to help eliminate skull asymmetry while the infant's head is growing rapidly (head circumference enlargement). Rather than aggressively shaping the skull, orthotic helmets protect the flats from pressure and help the head grow to push out the flats. Orthotic helmet treatment achieves correction three times faster and better than physiotherapy alone [1]. This treatment needs to be performed at a specialized medical institution for reasons such as cost/time requirements, applicable range, and side effects (inflammation, rash, pressure ulcer).

4.1 Start of Treatment

Starting as early as possible, before the skull deformity progresses to a severe degree, leads to greater improvements in deformity. In general, if the condition is as described above, it will start at 2–3 months after birth. For infants who have been followed up without physical therapy until the 3–4-month medical checkup, we will introduce them to a specialist early, considering that it takes approximately 2 weeks from ordering to wearing an orthotic helmet for orthotic treatment. If the ordered orthotic helmet cannot be worn on the specified date and time elapses, the deformation of the skull progresses further, creating a mismatch between the manufactured helmet and the skull deformity, and the corrective effect decreases. This is explained to the parents, and the data acquisition date for making the helmet is determined by calculating backward from the day when the child can visit the hospital.

4.2 Treatment Period and Indication of Completion

In severe cases, treatment is started at 4–5 months of age, and the average duration of wearing a helmet is about 6 months if the helmet is worn 23 h a day.

References

1. Fahrenkopf MP, Adams NS, Mann AR, Girotto JA. Deformational plagiocephaly. In: Kliegman RM, St Geme JW, editors. Nelson textbook of pediatrics 21st. Amsterdam: Elsevier; 2019. p. 3082–6.
2. Laughlin J, Luerssen TG, Dias MS, Committee on Practice and Ambulatory Medicine, Section on Neurological Surgery. Prevention and management of positional skull deformities in infants. Pediatrics. 2011;128:1236–41.
3. Back to Sleep, Tummy to Play. Health Children com. https://www.healthychildre n.org/English/ages-stages/baby/sleep/Pages/Back-to-Sleep-Tummy-to-Play.aspx. Accessed 31 Dec 2021.
4. Ditthakasem K, Kolar JC. Deformational Plagiocephaly: a review. Pediatr Nurs. 2017;43:59–64.
5. Tummy Time Activities. Health Children.com. https://www.healthychildren.org/English/ages-stages/baby/sleep/Pages/The-Importance-of-Tummy-Time.aspx.

Part III
Diagnosis and Treatment at Specialized Hospitals

Chapter 4
Basic Concepts for Diagnosing Cranial Deformity

Yasuo Aihara

1 Index of Cranial Deformity

In general, the anterior fontanelle closes around 7–15 months after birth, but there are cases in which even in healthy children, it is already close to closure at 4–5 months after birth. Conversely, compensatory enlargement of the head circumference for symptoms of increased intracranial pressure due to disease not only increases the tension of the anterior fontanelle but also allows diagnosis of dissection of the skull sutures by palpation.

In the cranial morphology (symmetry) examination, not only the shape of the head but also auricle position displacement, facial bone displacement, facial asymmetry, and mandibular displacement are confirmed. It is important to visually inspect and palpate the patient to check for neck and hip joint dislocations (the hip joints on the side opposite to the plagiocephaly tend to dislocate). Furthermore, it is necessary to discriminate premature cranial synostosis by referring to the patency of the anterior fontanelle and the presence or absence of trabecular bone formation on the suture line by palpating the anterior and posterior fontanelles, and the suture line of the skull at the time of health checkups for infants.

Y. Aihara (✉)
Department of Neurosurgery, Tokyo Women's Medical University, Tokyo, Japan
e-mail: yaihara@twmu.ac.jp

S. Kusuda et al. (eds.), *Handbook of Positional Plagiocephaly*,
https://doi.org/10.1007/978-981-97-9164-4_4

2 Cranial Deformity and SIDS

In the United States, in 1992, the American Academy of Pediatrics (AAP) recommended that infants sleep on their backs to prevent sudden infant death syndrome (SIDS) (the so-called Back to Sleep campaign). While the incidence of SIDS decreased, the incidence of cranial deformity increased.

In Japan, cranial deformity has not been considered a major problem until now, rather considered a self-limiting condition to return spontaneously with growth.

3 Premature Cranial Suture Synostosis

In premature cranial suture synostosis, a part of, multiple, and even sometimes all cranial sutures fuse early in the fetal period to 1 year of age, resulting in cranial deformity and secondary intracranial hypertension. Because of the complication of psychomotor developmental disorder associated with this condition, it is necessary to perform cranial correction surgery at an appropriate time. This is an important point for diagnosis.

Abnormal cranial suture fusion in infants can usually be verified by cranial X-ray or computed tomography scan. If no synostosis was found, many cases with severe cranial deformity which well exceeded congenital cranial synostosis in deformity degree were successfully treated without surgical procedures [1].

4 Positional Plagiocephaly

Positional plagiocephaly and its effects are not widely known, and there are no population-based studies on its frequency [2]. One problem faced is the wide variety of terms connoting this medical state. A partial list of terms used to refer to positional plagiocephaly is given in Table 4.1.

Table 4.1 Other terminology for positional plagiocephaly

• Benign positional molding
• Lambdoid plagiocephaly
* Lambda: Cranial measurement point where the lactate suture and the lambda suture meet
• Deformational plagiocephaly
• Occipital plagiocephaly
• Posterior plagiocephaly
* Characterized by partial thinning and softening of the skull, and widening of sutures and fontanelles
• Cranioscoliosis
• Dysmorphic calvarium

Further, some consider the general definition of positional plagiocephaly to be "the morphological change that affects normal tissue deformation and remodeling [3]." However, in general, brain growth and development in children with positional plagiocephaly are considered to be normal. A Dutch study that investigated positional preference among 7609 infants found that in the first month after birth, 8.2% of infants demonstrated a bias (i.e., many infants preferred either the left or right when changing their head position) [4]. However, in follow-up studies conducted until 6–8 months of age, 47% of infants developed asymmetric flattening of the occiput, while in 23% of infants, the condition had progressed to asymmetric flattening of the forehead. In addition, approximately 3% of infants were diagnosed with positional plagiocephaly, a severe form of deformation that requires surgical treatment [3].

In Japan, there is little awareness of the details of positional cranial deformation even among health-care workers. Although multiple case report studies on its effects on children and their prognoses are extremely limited [5], we will attempt to reference this research in the next chapter.

References

1. Argenta LC, David LR, Wilson JA, et al. An increase in infant cranial deformity with sleeping position. J Craniofac Surg. 1996;7(1):5–11.
2. Rekate HL. Occipital plagiocephaly: a critical review of the literature. J Neurosurg. 1998;89(1):24–30.
3. Graham JM Jr, Charman CE, Chaisson R, et al. Postnatal head deformation: anthropological observations and applications to the treatment of postnatal plagiocephaly, vol. 7. Proceedings of the Greenwood Genetic Center; 1988. p. 156–9.
4. Boere-Boonekamp MM, van der Linden-Kuiper LT. Positional preference: prevalence in infants and follow-up after two years. Pedatrics. 2001;107(2):339–43.
5. Aihara Y, Komatsu K, Dairoku H, et al. Cranial molding helmet therapy and establishment of practical criteria for management in Asian infant positional head deformity. Childs Nerv Syst. 2014;30(9):1499–509.

Chapter 5
Understanding Positional Plagiocephaly

Yasuo Aihara

1 Misunderstanding Caused by the Expression "Positional"

The most problematic interpretations of the term tend to stem from the usual expression "positional" plagiocephaly. This leads to a misunderstanding of social interpretation, leading to the association that cranial deformity is simply the result of lying down and can be remedied by evenly repositioning the child to relieve pressure on the flattened area. Moreover, for infants with positional plagiocephaly, repositioning and stretching are effective techniques in the early stages, before they can move around on their own. However, once the infant begins to roll over on its own, the effect is lost. This is because it is extremely difficult for infants and toddlers during the period of rolling over to stay still in a fixed place without considerable restraint.

However, the term "positional" is an oversimplification of not only prenatal factors but also postnatal factors that contribute to many cranial deformities. Tables 5.1 and 5.2 list many prenatal and postnatal factors involved in positional plagiocephaly.

Y. Aihara (✉)
Department of Neurosurgery, Tokyo Women's Medical University, Tokyo, Japan
e-mail: yaihara@twmu.ac.jp

S. Kusuda et al. (eds.), *Handbook of Positional Plagiocephaly*,
https://doi.org/10.1007/978-981-97-9164-4_5

Table 5.1 Prenatal factors for positional plagiocephaly

• Environment in the restrained uterus (pressure on the fetus)
• First birth
The width and shape of the uterus are particularly restricted during the first pregnancy
• Breech presentation
Even in cesarean births, the fetal head has a long head shape
It comes out pushing into the abdominal cavity of the mother
• Prolonged dystocia
The fetal head is pushed into the birth canal and comes out
• Multiple pregnancies
Develops deformative plagiocephaly due to narrow intrauterine space

Table 5.2 Postnatal factors of positional plagiocephaly

• Congenital muscular torticollis
Limited range of motion of the neck causes positional plagiocephaly. Positional plagiocephaly may also occur when the reduced ability to turn the deformed head results in inadequate or negative range of motion
• Weak muscle tone
Hypotonicity and weakness of the neck limit the range of neck extension and movement of the head from side to side. Continuous resting of the head in place causes cranial deformity and flattening. A misshapen head requires considerable effort to turn, causing loss of the developing neck muscle mechanics
• Long-term care in the NICU
Premature infants and infants under respiratory management are placed alternately on the right and left sides with intubation tubes and leads attached. The extremely soft preterm skull rapidly progresses to an abnormal long-cephalic (navicular) cranial shape. To prevent regurgitation of gastric contents, management in the right lateral decubitus position has increased, and there is a tendency for right occipital plagiocephaly. Some children discharged from the NICU do not have sufficient muscle strength and motor control to change their head position
• Abnormalities of the cervical spine
When combined with congenital structural abnormalities, it can cause an imbalance in the position of the head and neck, putting the infant's skull at risk of deformity
• Position for lying on the back
It tends to worsen the progression of deformation. Some parents have not been instructed that it is possible to provide "sprawl time" while the infant is awake
• Inadequate ossification
Preterm infants have softer skulls and are more susceptible to deformities than term infants
• Birth trauma
May be caused by forceps or vacuum delivery (e.g., cephalohematoma)
• Preterm infants
Delayed neuromotor development can lead to excessive cranial deformation of the occiput and forehead

2 Different Variants

Plagiocephaly is one element in a series of deformities. Other medical abnormalities may accompany this deformity and are directly or indirectly related to cranial deformity (Table 5.3).

Positional plagiocephaly is sometimes treated as a very mild condition that is simply flattening at the occipital region of the skull. However, the skull consists of several small bones, and deformation of one bone leads to deformation of the entire skull and abnormal arrangement of all connections and structures. Table 5.4 shows cranial asymmetry symptoms that are generally identified with positional plagiocephaly.

Infants with craniofacial asymmetry and torticollis may attempt to compensate for abnormal head structures with normal organ displacements, resulting in visual and vestibular deficits. Furthermore, orbital distortion can create sustained stress on the infraorbital muscles and nerves, resulting in sensorimotor disturbances.

Table 5.3 Direct and indirect effects of positional plagiocephaly

Direct	Indirect
• Facial deformation	• Positional deformation of the foot (end of the foot)
• Asymmetry of the mandible	• Dysplasia of deformed hips
• Congenital muscular torticollis or acquired muscular torticollis	• Infection of the middle ear (tympanic membrane)
• Abnormal eye position	• Migraine
• Deformation of the outer surface of the ear and abnormal left–right position	
• Orbital asymmetry that causes strabismus and other visual disturbances	
• Palpebral nasal folds on the side of the flat part	

Table 5.4 Cranial asymmetry symptoms equated with positional plagiocephaly

• Abnormal skull height
• Abnormal cranial width and spread
• Occipital flattening with plagiocephaly and ipsilateral forehead protrusion
• Excessive misalignment of ears
• Abnormal arrangement and asymmetry of the orbit
• Abnormal nose displacement (deviation), asymmetric cheek features, and ridges
• Abnormal jaw displacement (deviation)

3 Orthodontic Treatments for Cranial Deformity and Literature Reviews

Cranial orthotic treatment works directly on the 2 frontal, 2 parietal, 2 sphenoid, 2 temporal, and 1 occipital bone of the cranium. The direct transfer of force through the tissue of the brain indirectly affects the entire facial array (i.e., the cranium). The studies that report on the efficacy of cranial orthotic treatment are summarized below.

- Conclusion by Clarren et al. (1979) [1]: Cranial correction treatment is safe and effective for positional plagiocephaly.[.
- Conclusion by Rekate et al. (1998) [2]: Cranial correction therapy should be indicated for infants with positional plagiocephaly under 12 months of age who still have residual asymmetry despite attempted repositioning.
- Littlefield et al. (1999) [3]: Improvement in cranial deformity can be achieved with cranial orthotic treatment and is maintained after treatment.
- Kelly et al. (1999) [4]: The need for early orthotic intervention was confirmed. Asymmetry is exacerbated during periods of rapid cranial growth. The effectiveness of orthotic treatment diminishes in proportion to the reduced likelihood of regeneration due to cranial stiffness.[.
- Conclusion by Kelly et al. (1999) [5]: Complications associated with cranial asymmetry appear to be statistically related to plagiocephaly deformity.
- Joganic et al. (1995) [6]: Use of cranial correction therapy to enhance postoperative outcomes.
- Graham et al. (1988) [7]: We established the importance of early intervention in cranial orthotic treatment in terms of both the duration and outcome of the orthotic treatment program. The rate of shape change is related to brain growth and is more pronounced during the first 6 months of life than during early childhood. In a prospective study of 114 infants, 63 infants placed in their cribs and 51 treated with helmet correction showed significantly better results in occipitocranial symmetry.

4 Critical Stages of Development and Positional Plagiocephaly

The general concept of the course of positional plagiocephaly is that when infants develop the ability to engage in more significant activity, begin to roll over, and/or acquire a sitting position, the condition will naturally improve to some extent, so active treatment is unnecessary. This belief stems from a lack of understanding of the criteria for motor development and the consequences of sleeping on the back. Patterns of early motor neuron development are influenced by sleeping position. On average, it has been reported that in the case of lying on the back, the time to reach the critical stage of general motor nerves is later than in the case of lying on the stomach [8].

Before 1992, infants who were put to sleep on their stomach generally assumed various postures during the day and did not stay in the same position for a long time, so their head shapes were repaired in the first two to 3 months of life. While lying on one's back is now one of many positions, it delays the time when infants learn to control their head and torso by 4–6 weeks. In addition, it also interfered with the phenomenon of the natural course of the baby's head becoming round, which had been taken for granted until now.

However, to prevent SIDS, it is mandatory for the infant to sleep on the back.

5 Torticollis and Positional Plagiocephaly

Congenital muscular torticollis is a common neonatal musculoskeletal deformity that may be the result of and concomitant with positional plagiocephaly, or secondary torticollis causing positional plagiocephaly.

Binder et al. studied the long-term effects of torticollis and found that there are many cases of mild or moderate torticollis that were completely cured with early intervention but have persistent complex physical aspects of functional asymmetry [9].

References

1. Clarren SK, Smith DW, Hanson JW. Helmet treatment for plagiocephaly and congenital muscular torticollis. J Pediatr. 1979;94(1):43–6.
2. Rekate HL. Occipital plagiocephaly: a critical review of the literature. J Neurosurg. 1998;89(1):24–30.
3. Littlefield T, Pomatto J, Beals S, et al. Efficacy and stability of dynamic orthotic Cranioplasty: an eight-year investigation. Cleft Palate Craniofac J. 1999;36(2):127–30.
4. Kelly KM, Littlefield TR, Pomatto JK, et al. Importance of early recognition and treatment of deformational plagiocephaly with orthotic cranioplasty. Cleft Palate–Craniofacial J. 1999;36(2):127–30.
5. Kelly KM, Littlefield TR, Pomatto JK, et al. Cranial growth unrestricted during treatment of deformational plagiocephaly. Pediatr Neurosurg. 1999;30(4):193–9.
6. Joganic EF, Beals SP, Ripley J, et al. Enhancement of craniofacial reconstruction by dynamic orthotic cranioplasty. In: Proceedings of the VI Congress of the International Society of Craniofacial Surgery; 1995. p. 151–3.
7. Graham JM Jr, Charman CE, Chaisson R, et al. Postnatal head deformation: anthropological observations and applications to the treatment of postnatal plagiocephaly. In: Proceedings of the Greenwood Genetic Center, vol. 7; 1988. p. 156–9.
8. Davis BE, Moon RY, Sachs HC, et al. Effects of sleep position on infant motor development. Pediatrics. 1998;102(5):1135–40.
9. Binder H, Eng GD, Gaiser JF, et al. Congenital muscular torticollis: results of conservative management with long-term follow-up in 85 cases. Arch Phys Med Rehabil. 1987;68(4):222–5.

Chapter 6
Differential Diagnosis

Yasuo Aihara

1 Hydrocephalus

It is necessary to distinguish hydrocephalus as a representative disease from other congenital disorders. Hydrocephalus is difficult to definitively diagnose by measuring the head circumference at a single point in time. If the patient deviates significantly from the growth curve of the head circumference over time, the tension of the fontanelle is higher than normal and is accompanied by moodiness, which may lead to psychomotor development disorder, requiring diagnosis. However, until infancy, head circumference enlargement compensates for intracranial hypertension. Therefore, it is sometimes noticed in episodes such as "It became difficult to pass their head through when wearing clothes" and "Their hat became tighter in an abnormally short time, and they can't wear it anymore."

Causes of hydrocephalus include congenital intracranial anomalies (arachnoid cysts), brain tumors, intracranial hemorrhages such as subependymal hemorrhage, and cerebrospinal fluid malabsorption secondary to meningitis. Others include genetic and hormonal abnormalities, secondary subdural hematoma, and subdural edema from trauma. Cranial ultrasonography is useful in infancy, including the neonatal period, but the definitive diagnosis is made by plain X-ray imaging for enlarged skull suture dissection and CT/magnetic resonance imaging.

Y. Aihara (✉)
Department of Neurosurgery, Tokyo Women's Medical University, Tokyo, Japan
e-mail: yaihara@twmu.ac.jp

S. Kusuda et al. (eds.), *Handbook of Positional Plagiocephaly*,
https://doi.org/10.1007/978-981-97-9164-4_6

2 Premature Cranial Suture Synostosis

Conversely, in patients with poor head circumference growth, it is possible to make a primary diagnosis as screening by inspection and palpation based on the diagnostic criteria for cranial deformity used overseas when examining cranial deformity. However, it is necessary to consider the mechanism of normal head growth and its growth curve (Fig. 6.1).

- Possibility of pathological cranial deformity (premature cranial suture synostosis) and positional cranial deformity due to orientation in the same case.
- In the case of premature synostosis of all sutures, microcephaly without any asymmetry (head circumference of 3 percentile value or less).

If it is difficult to make a diagnosis only by palpation of the skull, a cephalometric X-ray (frontal, lateral, and Towne views) will be performed to determine the patency of the anterior fontanelle, the disconnection of the suture line, and the presence or absence of finger impressions. Surgical craniofacial osteoplasty should be performed before the age of 1 year in cases of premature cranial suture synostosis with symptoms of increased intracranial pressure, such as digital marking on imaging.

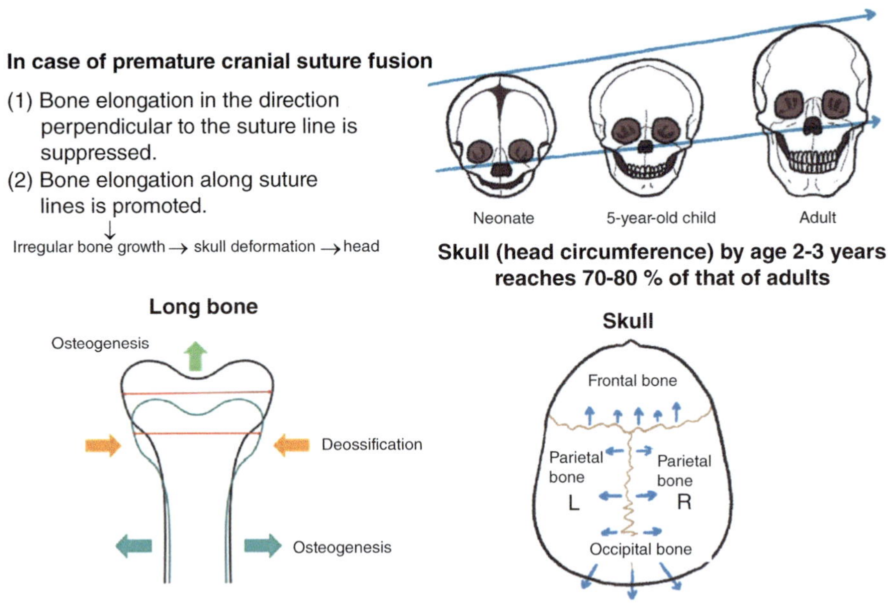

Fig. 6.1 Basic principle of head circumference growth. Long bones grow mainly longitudinally of the diaphysis, whereas skulls grow vertically from the skull sutures. (©Nabeco)

3 Definitive Diagnosis after Differential Diagnosis

For severe positional cranial deformity in infants, many cases can be treated with orthotic helmet treatment without surgery if the sutures are patent (at a young age before the closure of the great fontanelle). To make a definitive diagnosis, a head X-ray examination is necessary, but starting with palpation of the anterior fontanelle, palpating the suture line of the occipital and plagiocephaly, and in the case of positional plagiocephaly, the plagiocephalic part should be palpated. It is important to ascertain whether there is a forehead side displacement that coincides with the cranial side. If the forehead on the ipsilateral side of the plagiocephaly is displaced posteriorly, premature synostosis of the forehead should be suspected (Figs. 6.2, 6.3 and 6.4).

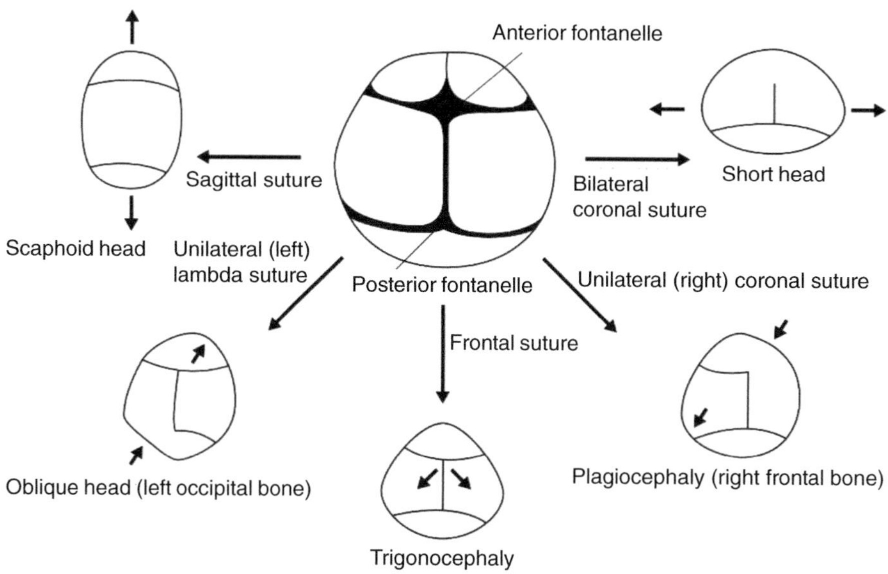

Fig. 6.2 Cranial deformity associated with early synostosis of cranial sutures. Skull shape alone is difficult to distinguish from the positional cranial deformity. (©Nabeco)

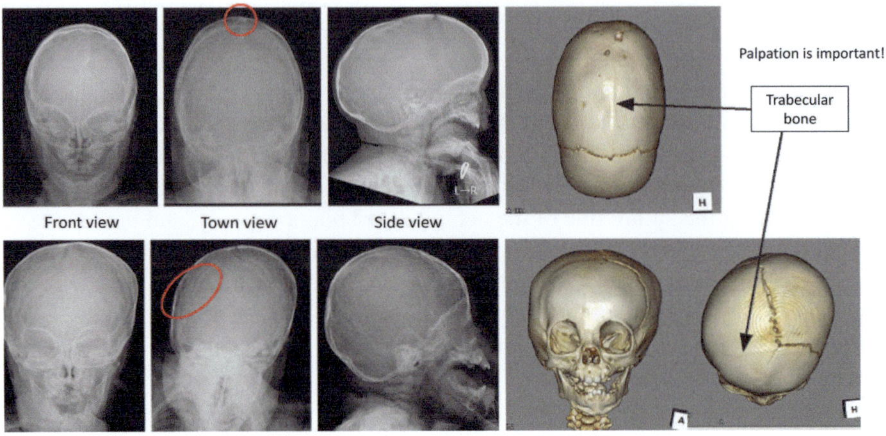

Fig. 6.4 Cranial X-ray and three-dimensional (3D) CT bone findings of premature cranial suture synostosis. Fusion is suspected on the X-ray (inside the red frame), and a definitive diagnosis is made with 3D CT bone. Palpation of the trabecular bone at suture fusions is also a very important finding. (©Nabeco)

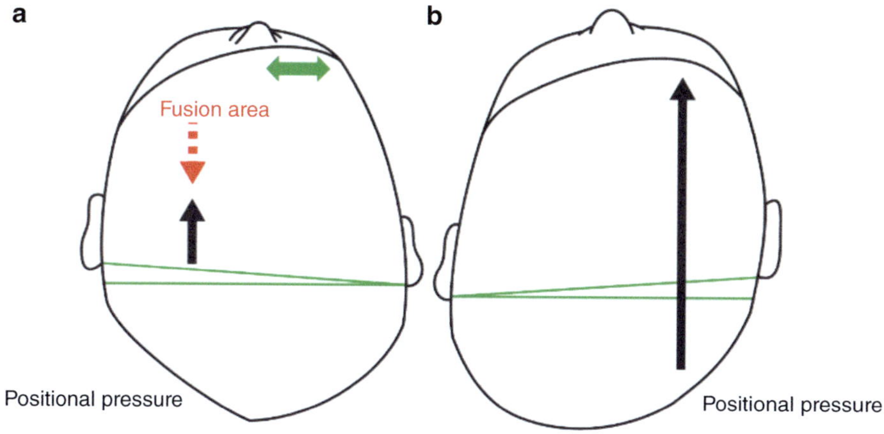

Fig. 6.3 Differentiation between premature cranial suture synostosis and positional plagiocephaly. (**a**) A case of complication of premature cranial suture synostosis (left coronal suture) and positional plagiocephaly (left human letter suture). The left occipital region is deformed under the influence of gravity from lying down, and the left side of the auricle moves forward accordingly. When the left coronary suture is prematurely fused, the impression is that the left forehead is pulled backward, but sometimes it interferes with the pressure displacement findings of the left forehead due to positional plagiocephaly, giving the impression that there is no displacement. Simultaneously, the right forehead on the unaffected side appears to protrude forward, but it is not displaced. (**b**) Right occipital positional plagiocephaly. The right occipital region is deformed under the influence of gravity, and the auricle position moves forward on the right side. As a feature here, the right forehead on the ipsilateral side protrudes forward in conjunction with pressure from the occipital region. (©Nabeco)

Chapter 7
Whole Body Effects of Cranial Deformity

Yasuo Aihara

1 First, Understanding "Displacement"

In general, many of the families who visit the clinic because they are worried about the cranial deformity of their child (infant) are concerned about the "appearance of cranial shape from the parietal side."

At this time, it is important to explain the mechanism of cranial deformation using a skull model. The "cranium," which is the subject of medical treatment, is a name that includes all of the temporomandibular joint, the base of the skull (including the auricle, external auditory canal, pyramidal bone, temporomandibular joint, etc.), and frontal, temporal, and parietal bones. To reiterate, the purpose of cranial correction is not to improve the cosmetic appearance (symmetry). Even if the cranial deformity is caused by head position preference, it is necessary to understand that this is a pathological condition in which the skull is "displaced" relative to the skull base itself around the centerline (Fig. 7.1).

2 Complications Secondary to "Displacement"

If the cranial deformation sets in without correction, the complication rate of otitis media due to auricle (pyramidal bone, external auditory canal deformation) displacement and occlusion disorder due to temporomandibular joint displacement increases. In addition, once children can walk, it tends to affect the whole trunk balance. At the cranial deformity outpatient clinic, the parents themselves suffered

---

Y. Aihara (✉)
Department of Neurosurgery, Tokyo Women's Medical University, Tokyo, Japan
e-mail: yaihara@twmu.ac.jp

S. Kusuda et al. (eds.), *Handbook of Positional Plagiocephaly*,
https://doi.org/10.1007/978-981-97-9164-4_7

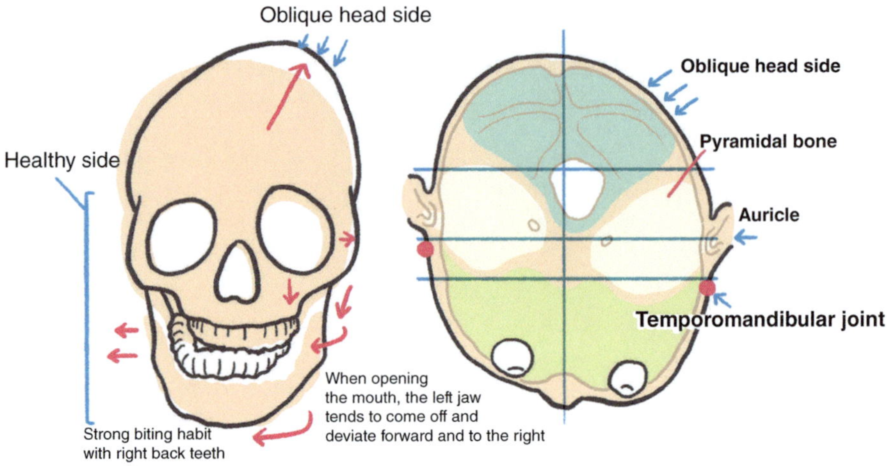

Fig. 7.1 Skull misalignment. Improving skull symmetry is not a treatment goal. Improving deformations at the base of the skull (pyramidal bone, anterior/middle/posterior skull), external auditory canal, and temporomandibular joint area results in an improvement of symmetry ratio. (©Nabeco)

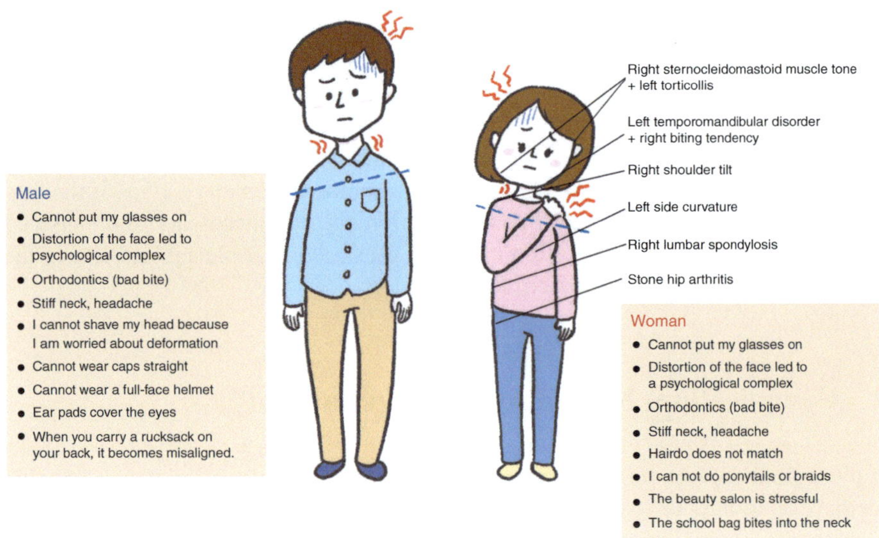

Fig. 7.2 Opportunity for visiting a cranial deformity outpatient clinic. In many cases, the parents themselves suffered severe cranial deformity. (©Nabeco)

from secondary temporomandibular disorders, torticollis, migraines, stiff shoulders, scoliosis, low back pain, and so on. Many patients complain that they visited the hospital out of fear that they would suffer from similar symptoms in the future (Fig. 7.2).

Chapter 8
Importance of Infant Health Checkup in Cranial Deformity

Yasuo Aihara

1 Importance of 1-Month Checkup

It is no exaggeration to say that the point of contact for cranial health checkups and screening are all places for general infant health checkups. In the major premise of early diagnosis and early intervention, it is very important to diagnose cranial deformity, especially the rate of cranial deformity in 1-month-old health checkup. However, due to the health checkup system, 1-month checkup is not necessarily confirmed by a pediatrician. Information sharing is essential.

2 Provision of Information on Optimal Orthotic Treatment Starting Age

The spontaneous positional cranial deformity is unlikely to correct spontaneously during later stages of growth once it progresses to moderate or severe deformity from the neonatal period to the first 2–3 months of age. This should be borne in mind. In addition, it is necessary to explain options for cranial deformity orthotic treatment and the optimal age for starting orthotic treatment (2–3 months after birth) to families at infant health checkups.

Y. Aihara (✉)
Department of Neurosurgery, Tokyo Women's Medical University, Tokyo, Japan
e-mail: yaihara@twmu.ac.jp

S. Kusuda et al. (eds.), *Handbook of Positional Plagiocephaly*,
https://doi.org/10.1007/978-981-97-9164-4_8

Chapter 9
Points of Medical Interview and Examination in Cranial Deformity

Yasuo Aihara

1 Collecting Information from Both Genetic and Environmental Perspectives

In infant health checkups, there are two points that families want to confirm with a doctor regarding the cranial deformation of their child as shown in Fig. 9.1

1. "What is the degree of skull deformation?"
2. "Is it okay to wait and see how this deformation is? Will it improve naturally?"

When examining the actual cranial deformity, it is necessary to check the head growth curve of the older brothers and sisters from the second child onward, referring to the parents' head circumference growth trends in the *Maternal and Child Health Handbook*. It is important to palpate and confirm the cranial shape. General expressions such as the size of the skull (large face, small face), face length, and "bee-likeness" have familial genetic predispositions, but positional cranial deformity is a change over time from birth. Carefully explain that environmental factors are more important than genetic predisposition.

2 Listen to Parents' Concerns

When doctors ask parents about cranial deformity, it is important to reach out about the following things: "Does your baby always sleep facing one side?" "Are you worried about that orientational preference?" "Are you worried about the deformation of the head shape due to orientational preference?" As a result, parents can be

Y. Aihara (✉)
Department of Neurosurgery, Tokyo Women's Medical University, Tokyo, Japan
e-mail: yaihara@twmu.ac.jp

S. Kusuda et al. (eds.), *Handbook of Positional Plagiocephaly*,
https://doi.org/10.1007/978-981-97-9164-4_9

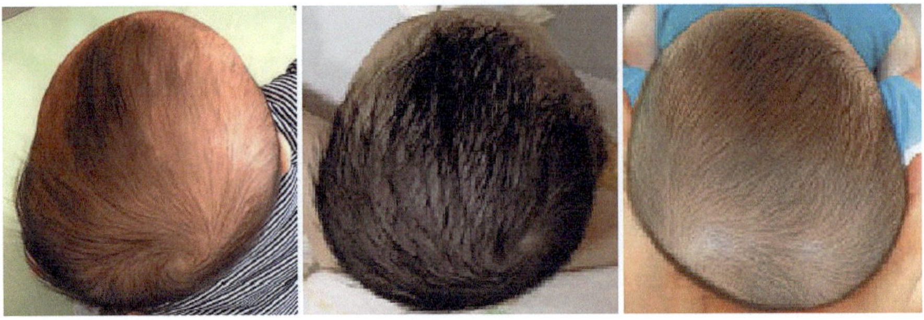

Fig. 9.1 Example of cranial deformity consulted during health checkups for infants. (©Nabeco)

relieved that their worries about "orientation" and "cranial deformity" are nothing special, and doctors can create an environment in which parents can easily disclose their worries about cranial deformity at the time of examination.

Most importantly, as health-care professionals, it is crucial to ensure that parenting errors do not cause cranial deformities. It is not uncommon for mothers to come to the hospital in a state of depression, believing that it is their fault that their child's skull has been deformed. Suppose there are no special secondary episodes (traumatic torticollis, cephalohematoma, etc.) at the time of birth, in that case, the head orientation is almost determined in the prenatal period, and the "direction of the orientation itself" is intentional. Explain that it is difficult to change.

Conversely, it is also possible to explain that it is extremely difficult to be "naturally corrected" the cranial deformity that is caused by facing positions and has become severe to a certain degree or more at 2 months after birth, during the subsequent growth process.

3 Questionnaire and Diagnosis/Classification

Ask the following ten questions.

1. How many children do you have? (Including single or multiple births).
2. How many weeks long was your pregnancy? (Calculation of corrected age): Simultaneously, compare and confirm the patency of the great fontanelle by palpation.
3. Since when have you been concerned about cranial deformity?
4. Which family member is most concerned about the deformity? (father, mother, grandparents, etc.)
5. When was the first time you consulted with a health-care professional?
6. Which department did you consult with? Or have you consulted a midwife?
7. What kind of instruction did you receive at that time?
8. Are there any medical workers among your parents or relatives? What do you think about the possibility of natural correction?

9. What kind of efforts have you made to date for cranial correction? What are the results?
10. Have your parents (and grandparents if they are present) been aware of any complexes regarding "cranial deformity" in your life so far? It is useful to diagnose the cranial morphology of both parents by palpation.

Using diagnostic criteria based on palpation makes it possible to make a diagnosis sufficiently without a measuring device.

4 Actual Examination

At the time of examination, the examining physician places the patient's head on both knees so that the parietal side of the patient's head can be easily seen by the facing family member (Fig. 9.2). Attaching a stretchable medical net to the head makes the outline of the skull clear, as shown in Fig. 9.3.

1. Displacement of auricle position.
2. Displacement of frontal protrusion on plagiocephaly side.
3. Displacement of the mandible.

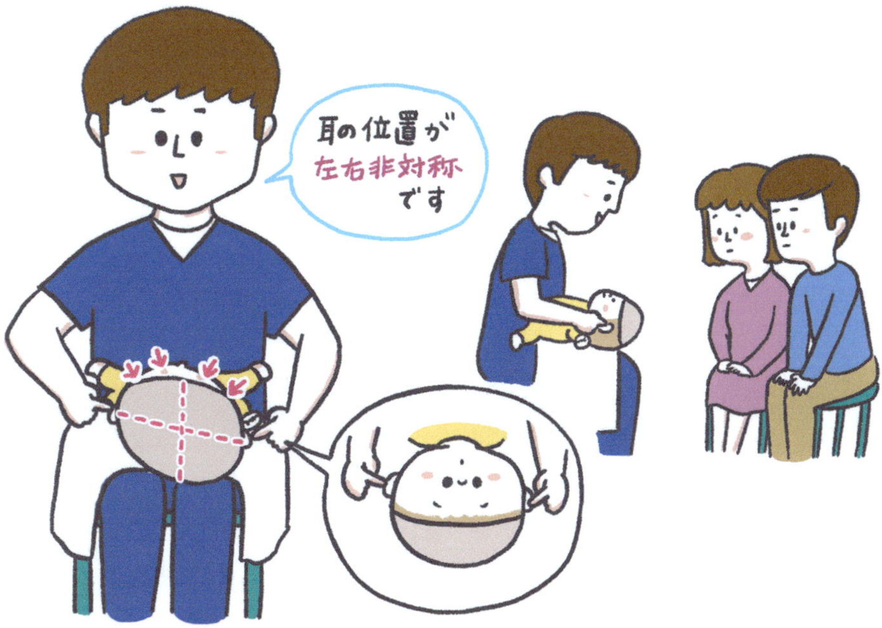

Palpation during examination (1) Confirmation of displacement of auricle position

Fig. 9.2 Palpation during examination: (1) Confirmation of displacement of auricle position. (©Nabeco)

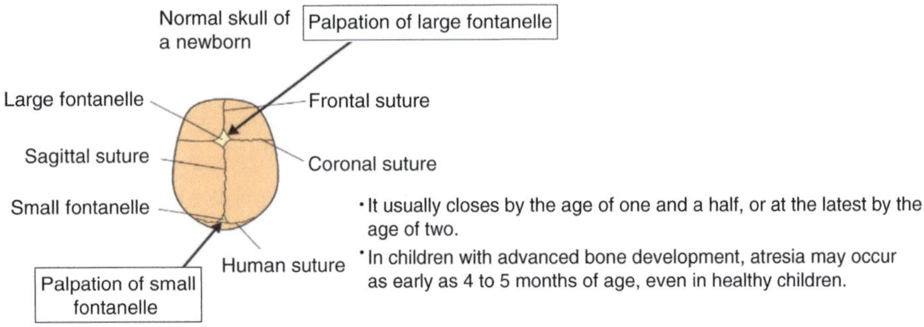

Fig. 9.3 Palpation during examination: (2) Check the patency of the large and small fontanels. (©Nabeco)

It is very helpful to explain to the family, pointing to the displacement.

If the auricle position is not displaced, it is class 1. If the auricle position is displaced by 1 cm (about one finger) or more, it is class 2. If there is facial (forehead) bone displacement, it is class 3. It is important to visually explain the presence of jawbone displacement, indicating that it is class 4.

If there are risk factors for developing cranial deformities such as low birth weight, torticollis, cephalohematoma, hip dislocation, hydrocephalus, premature synostosis, or multiple births, the class 5 deformity will not be corrected spontaneously and this outcome should be explained to their parents.

Chapter 10
Diagnosis Based on Cranial Deformation Measurements

Yasuo Aihara

1 Method for Calculating Cranial Deformity (CA)

To diagnose cranial deformity accurately and objectively, cranial asymmetry (CA) is calculated after cranial morphology is measured using a 3D laser scanner. However, the drawback of this diagnostic method is that it can only be performed using a 3D scanner. In addition, the auricle position displacement rate is not reflected in the deformation rate in this measurement method.

2 Screening Using the Application Software

Conversely, a screening method using a cranial deformation app is currently being developed (Fig. 10.1). However, it is important to recognize that the measurement of the cranial deformation app is an evaluation of a deformed plane. Cranial deformation is displacement/deformation in three dimensions, so it must be envisaged to evaluate the deformation rate as the entire skull. In clinical settings, there are cases in which even the most severe ones have slight auricle displacement in the assessment of CA and cranial vault asymmetry index (CVAI). Conversely, we experience very strong auricle displacement cases even if CA and CVAI rates are mild (Fig. 10.2).

Y. Aihara (✉)
Department of Neurosurgery, Tokyo Women's Medical University, Tokyo, Japan
e-mail: yaihara@twmu.ac.jp

S. Kusuda et al. (eds.), *Handbook of Positional Plagiocephaly*,
https://doi.org/10.1007/978-981-97-9164-4_10

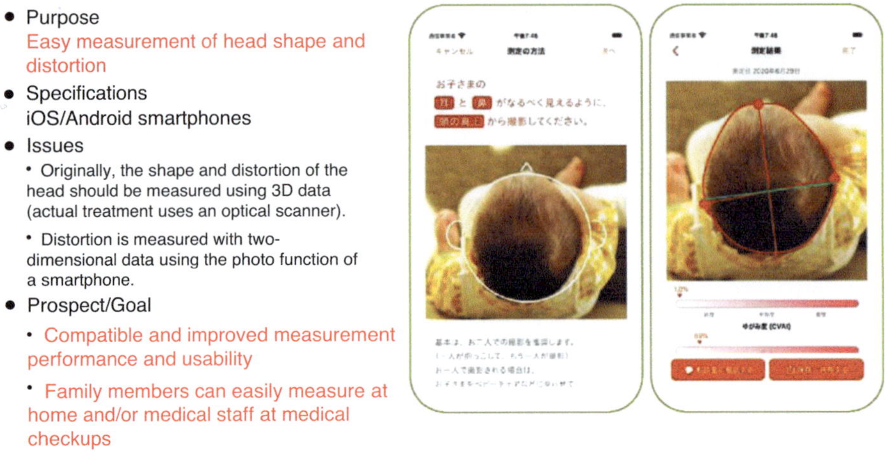

Fig. 10.1 Baby's head shape measurement app. (©Nabeco)

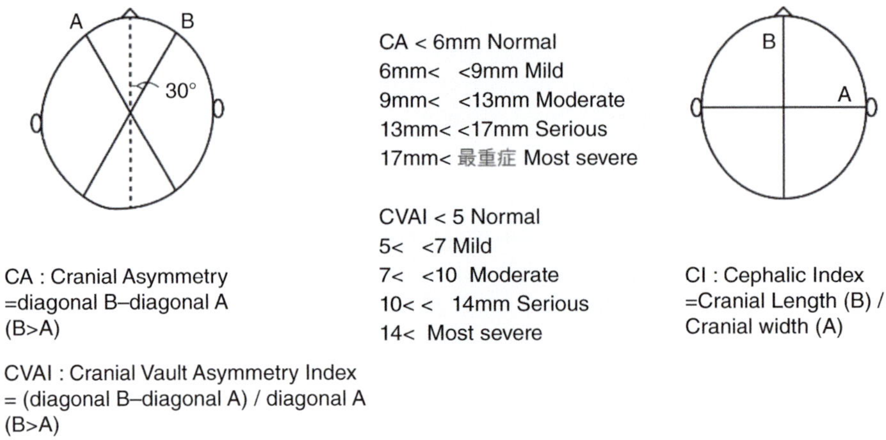

Fig. 10.2 Cranial deformation rate measurement method. (©Nabeco)

There are no clear criteria for diagnosing brachycephaly, even though the grading of plagiocephaly is defined. For cranial deformity in infants originating from Western countries (slightly long head), cephalic index (CI, determined by cranial length (B)/cranial width [A]) >120 is often used as a diagnostic index, but for Japanese (Asians), an index of >100 should be considered (Fig. 10.3).

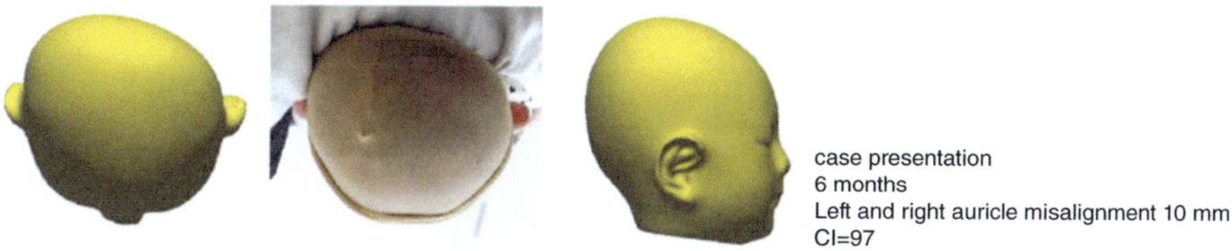

Fig. 10.3 Evaluation by CI (cephalic index)

Chapter 11
Expected Treatment Effect

Yasuo Aihara

1 How to Answer Questions About Treatment Efficacy?

It is expected that it will be necessary for the future to score the classifications shown in (p. 64) in more detail. Furthermore, in the future, it is necessary to consider the correction effect (expected value) instead of just the plagiocephaly rate for diagnosis. This is because conventional cranial deformity diagnosis has no "correction effect rate (prediction rate)." In the actual clinical setting of orthotic treatment, there are many questions from families, such as "What degree of orthotic effect can be expected when orthotic helmet treatment is performed?" However, the existing cranial deformity rate does not have a classification of indications for orthotic helmet treatment according to the patency of the great fontanelle and the presence or absence of complications.

It is also necessary to understand that "head circumference enlargement" (growth) is a very important factor in the treatment effect.

2 The Patency Rate of the Anterior Fontanelle Is an Important Indicator

In the future, it is desirable to use the expected value of the correction effect as an index by scoring in more detail, for example, as shown below, but the period of wearing the correction helmet, the expansion rate of the head circumference, and the closing time of the anterior fontanelle are unknown. Since there are many factors related to this, further investigation is considered necessary.

Y. Aihara (✉)
Department of Neurosurgery, Tokyo Women's Medical University, Tokyo, Japan
e-mail: yaihara@twmu.ac.jp

S. Kusuda et al. (eds.), *Handbook of Positional Plagiocephaly*,
https://doi.org/10.1007/978-981-97-9164-4_11

●Calculation image of the expected value of the correction effect.

Deformation rate class () + Corrected age () + Great fontanelle patency () + Complications () = () points.

() points - () point = Expected correction value Class 1 target possible.

() point - () points = Great correction effect can be expected, but difficult up to Class 1.

() point - () = Corrective effect can be expected, but about Class 1 improvement.

It is important to evaluate the patency of the anterior fontanelle at the time of initial examination in the clinical examination of the skull. Since "bone age" is generally used to evaluate normal ossification such as osteomalacia, the expression "patency" is used. Even among children of the same age, the patency of the anterior fontanelle varies greatly among individuals. Therefore, children with a low patency are expected to have a poor correction effect even at a young age, while children with a high patency are expected to have a correction effect even at an older age. Considering this possibility, in the future, it will be necessary to quantify and classify the anterior fontanelle's patency.

Chapter 12
Feedback from Specialty Medical Institutions

Yasuo Aihara

1 When Early Intervention Is Required

A rapid head enlargement accompanied by symptoms of increased intracranial pressure indicates early therapeutic intervention based on a definitive diagnosis by imaging diagnosis at a specialized medical institution. Even in infants with cranial deformity, progressive craniofacial bone deformation in the course of follow-up demands early treatment (surgical/orthotic) or intervention based on definitive diagnosis by images in cases with enlargement of the head circumference.

2 For Follow-Up

Even though the head circumference exceeds the standard curve line, just follow-up is recommended if there are following findings: no abnormality in palpation of head, the head enlargement along the standard curve, good general condition, large head circumferences of siblings and parents, and no pathological characteristic other than enlarged head circumference.

Furthermore, if the cranial deformity is mild and there is no abnormality in palpation, follow-up is also possible.

Y. Aihara (✉)
Department of Neurosurgery, Tokyo Women's Medical University, Tokyo, Japan
e-mail: yaihara@twmu.ac.jp

S. Kusuda et al. (eds.), *Handbook of Positional Plagiocephaly*,
https://doi.org/10.1007/978-981-97-9164-4_12

3 If Head Circumference Growth Is Small

If there is no enlargement of the head circumference, but rather the growth of the head circumference is small, it is necessary to differentiate all suture premature synostosis (high cranial symmetry rate, small head circumference) among premature cranial suture synostosis.

4 When Natural Correction Is Difficult

The degree of positional plagiocephaly is class 3 or higher, regardless of age, and conveys the fact that it already belongs to the group of deformities that are difficult to correct naturally (Fig. 12.1). It is also explained that there are options that can be considered as part of individuality and options for orthotic helmet treatment and that there are adaptation restrictions according to the child's age for orthotic helmet treatment.

Since the suitability for orthotic helmet treatment cannot be determined based on age alone, early consultation is recommended (the optimal age for starting orthotic helmet treatment is 2–3 months after birth).

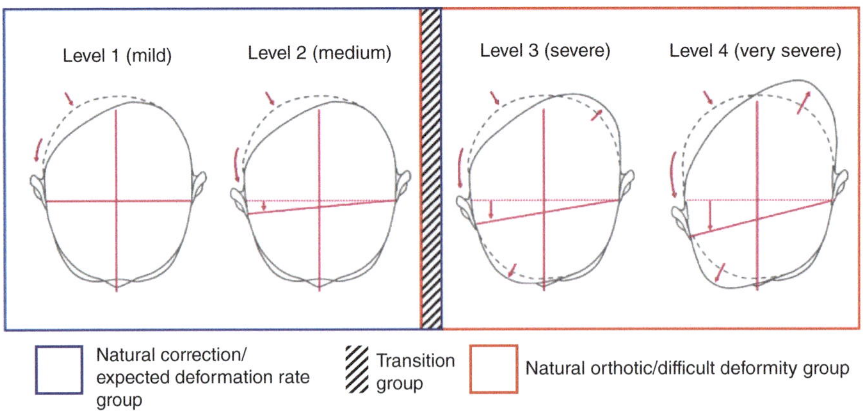

Fig. 12.1 Levels where natural correction can be expected and levels where it is difficult. (©Nabeco)

Chapter 13
Mechanisms of Cranial Orthotic Treatment and Inner Layer Structure of the Orthotic Helmet

Yasuo Aihara

Three types of orthotic helmets have been introduced in Japan, each with a different structure. In this handbook, the structure and therapeutic mechanism of Aimet® (manufactured by the Japan Medical Company) is explained.

1 Return the “Misalignment” to the Correct Position

The pathology of cranial deformity is mainly caused from the “deviation” of the central axis of the skull. Cranial orthotic treatment aims at returning this “displacement” to its original (before deformation) anatomically correct position. Therefore, the inner layer structure of the orthotic helmet is designed to prevent deterioration of the cranial deformity on the long axis side that has already been displaced and deformed, and simultaneously induce the growth of the skull on the plagiocephaly side (Fig. 13.1).

Therefore, when wearing an orthotic helmet, the long axis in the case of deformed plagiocephaly and the left and right horizontal axes in the case of brachycephaly are firmly held so that the deformation does not progress or become more severe than at present.

Y. Aihara (✉)
Department of Neurosurgery, Tokyo Women’s Medical University, Tokyo, Japan
e-mail: yaihara@twmu.ac.jp

S. Kusuda et al. (eds.), *Handbook of Positional Plagiocephaly*,
https://doi.org/10.1007/978-981-97-9164-4_13

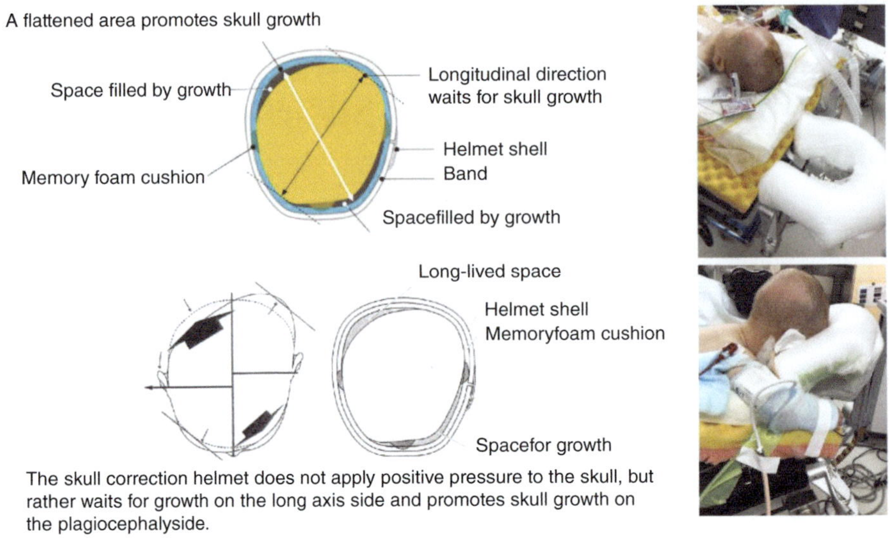

Fig. 13.1 Molding helmet correction mechanism and inner layer structure. The low-resilience material was developed based on the idea of a horseshoe cushion used during long craniotomy surgery for children. (©Nabeco)

2 Introduction of Low-Resilience Materials to Prevent Skin Problems

Infants who are the target of orthotic helmet treatment have fixed their sleeping preference on the flat surface of plagiocephaly and short heads until then, so all the weight of the skull is applied to the sharp deformed skull parts like the edge of a boat (Fig. 13.2: ● part). Therefore, paying attention to skin problems besides plagiocephaly is required after wearing an orthotic helmet. Based on the skin condition, the wearing time can be extended gradually.

Aimet® is composed of a special low-resilience cushion, and by holding the deformed skull with a "surface" rather than a "point," it reduces the frequency of skin troubles during the treatment. This idea originated in the development of a cushion horseshoe, which is used in the field of pediatric neurosurgery to hold the craniofacial during long-term craniotomy and prevent pressure ulcers during surgery (Fig. 13.1, right end).

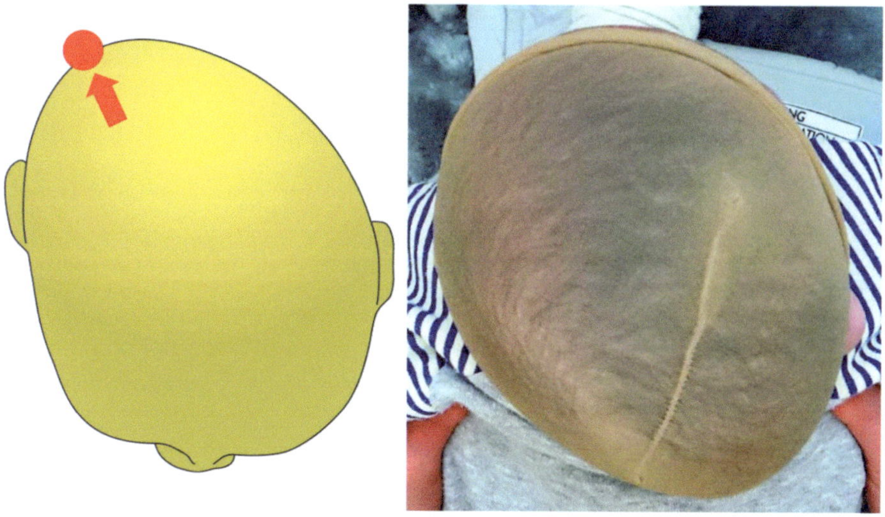

Fig. 13.2 Example of plagiocephaly. Class 4, 6 months (auricular position displacement 29 mm). (©Nabeco)

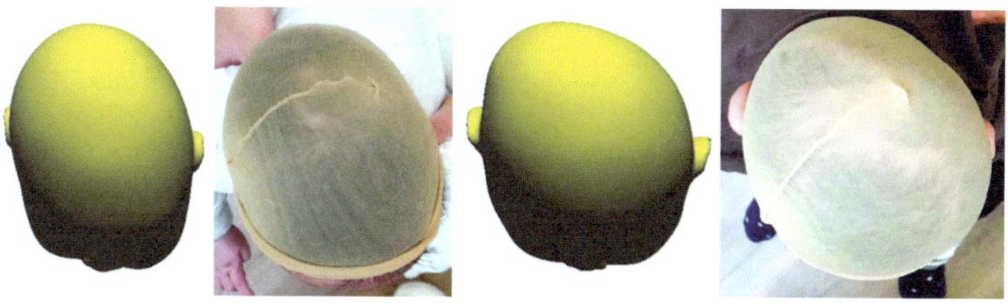

Fig. 13.3 Percentage of plagiocephaly and long head. Long-head plagiocephaly inevitably has a larger plagiocephaly area and is more difficult to correct naturally than short-head plagiocephaly

3 Setting the Offset Value According to the Deformation Pattern

For the same type of plagiocephaly, long-cephalic plagiocephaly tends to be more difficult to correct spontaneously than short-cephalic plagiocephaly. This is because the plagiocephaly area is inevitably large, making it difficult to change the head position (Fig. 13.3). At the first visit, it is important to confirm not only the severity of the plagiocephaly deformity and the displacement of the auricle but also the cranial length of the patient's cranial shape. It is also crucial to set the offset value of the inner layer of the helmet according to each cranial deformation pattern.

Chapter 14
Practice of Orthotic Helmet Wearing

Yasuo Aihara

1 Treatment Period and Wearing Time per Day

The duration of treatment with an orthotic helmet is up to 6 months as a guideline. However, there are no strict limits if the doctor performs regular checkups and is safely sizing considering the increased head circumference.

The wearing time per day is 23 h except for bathing. However, although it depends on when the infant starts wearing it, it is often difficult to wear it more than 23 h a day. During breastfeeding (5–6 times a day, 15–20 min each time: about 2 h in total), take off the orthotic helmet and give your child a break.

2 Pay Attention to Increased Perspiration and Core Temperature

Attention should be paid to the fact that heat builds up when wearing a helmet and the temperature of the trunk tends to rise because the helmet attachment surface is large relative to the total body surface area of the child. It is also necessary not to let them wear excessive clothing, not to raise the room temperature too much, and not to spend a long time wearing a helmet on a floor heater, hot carpet, and so on.

Always infants sweat more when wearing a helmet. In the group that starts orthotic treatment in autumn and winter, the amount of sweating may decrease even after long-term wearing due to the temperature drop, but in the group that starts orthotic treatment in spring and summer, the amount of sweat cannot decrease easily. Therefore, it is good to cool the scalp with cold towels during breaks. In

Y. Aihara (✉)
Department of Neurosurgery, Tokyo Women's Medical University, Tokyo, Japan
e-mail: yaihara@twmu.ac.jp

S. Kusuda et al. (eds.), *Handbook of Positional Plagiocephaly*,
https://doi.org/10.1007/978-981-97-9164-4_14

addition, if the child is getting older and scratching its head with its nails while it is not wearing an orthotic helmet, cut the nails short and use mittens (long socks are also useful) on both hands, teaching them as appropriate.

3 What to Do If Your Child Dislikes Orthotic Helmets

Conversely, if orthotic helmet treatment is started at its upper age limit, boys tend to remove their orthotic helmets at about 7 months of age, and girls at 9 months of age. As a result, many parents find it difficult to prolong treatment duration, causing them to worry. When starting orthotic treatment with a helmet at an older age, parents should be advised in advance that getting their child to wear a helmet during the day is likely to be difficult and that they should aim to wear a helmet for around 15 h a day, mainly during sleeping hours.

When children frequently take off their helmets, some parents try to apply a chin strap or a submandibular band for secure wearing. However, these extra bands must be removed because of the concern of suffocation.

3.1 [Trivia] Cosmetics Versus Reshaping

The American Medical Federation defines cosmetic procedures as "altering the normal structures of the body to enhance appearance." Reconstructive procedures, however, are defined as "procedures intended to promote the functioning of, or return to normal, abnormal structures of the body."

Children with craniofacial asymmetry and torticollis may attempt to compensate for abnormal head structures with a displacement of normal organs, resulting in visual and vestibular deficits. In addition, orbital distortion can create sustained stress on the infraorbital muscles and nerves, resulting in sensorimotor deficits.

Orthotic helmet treatment works directly on the frontal, parietal, sphenoid, temporal, and occipital bones. The direct transfer of force through the tissues of the brain indirectly affects the entire craniofacial array. Through orthotic helmet treatment, long-term auditory, visual, and jaw motor dysfunction can be avoided by returning the base of the skull, the cranial vault, the distance between the orbit and the outer ear, and the cranial and facial bones to their normal alignment.

Chapter 15
Pathological Disease Groups

Yasuo Aihara

1 Hydrocephalus (Indwelling Ventricular-Peritoneal Shunt Valve)

Neonatal/infantile onset hydrocephalus is complicated by rapid head circumference enlargement. Therefore, a pediatric neurosurgeon should perform a ventricular-abdominal shunt to control intracranial pressure.

Aimet R is made of a low-resilience cushioning material. Even in cases where a ventricle-peritoneal shunt circuit system is indwelled, it is possible to safely wear the shunt circuit by considering the location where the shunt circuit is buried. In addition, when the ossification of the skull is slow after a ventricular-peritoneal shunt indwelled, and the head circumference enlargement is difficult to control even with the lowest pressure setting, the orthotic helmet can serve as a virtual skull. It prevents abnormal head circumference enlargement without interfering with normal cranial growth, controls intracranial pressure, and waits for cranial ossification (Fig. 15.1a, b).

2 Premature Cranial Suture Synostosis

In the case of mild partial suture premature synostosis, improvement effects can be observed with orthotic helmet treatment alone without surgical osteoplasty. However, judgment by a specialist is required regarding indications for orthotic helmet treatment for early synostoses, such as the degree of suture fusion and evaluation of increased intracranial pressure. In general, an orthotic helmet is worn to

Y. Aihara (✉)
Department of Neurosurgery, Tokyo Women's Medical University, Tokyo, Japan
e-mail: yaihara@twmu.ac.jp

S. Kusuda et al. (eds.), *Handbook of Positional Plagiocephaly*,
https://doi.org/10.1007/978-981-97-9164-4_15

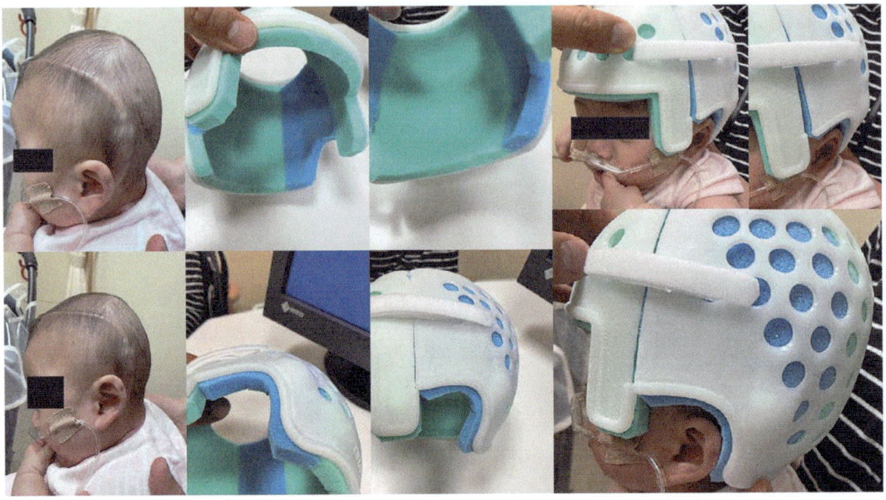

Fig. 15.1 (**a**) Fitting a corrective helmet to a child with hydrocephalus. (**b**) Head circumference change and cranial deformity in refractory hydrocephalus. Even with a shunt, head circumference enlargement continues due to insufficient ossification of the skull

support the surgical plastic effect as well as to prevent re-deformation after surgical cranioplasty. At that time, it is necessary to design an accurate orthotic helmet inner layer line considering the position of the bone extender after osteoplasty (Fig. 15.2a, b).

3 Retinopathy of Prematurity

Infants requiring long-term management in the NICU, such as low birth weight infants, are known to have a high cranial deformity rate. Such children also have a high complication rate of retinopathy of prematurity and need to wear corrective spectacles at an early stage. If an orthotic helmet is attached to a deformed cranium and the inner and outer layer structures of the helmet are used, it is possible to fix the corrective glasses more stably during infancy (Fig. 15.3).

4 Wearing a Continuous Positive Airway Pressure Mask

Infant patients with laryngomalacia and other conditions requiring continuous positive airway pressure (CPAP) at home tend to have a high cranial deformity rate because they inevitably spend a considerable amount of time in the recumbent position. In addition, there are several types of CPAP, and it is necessary to wear a mask

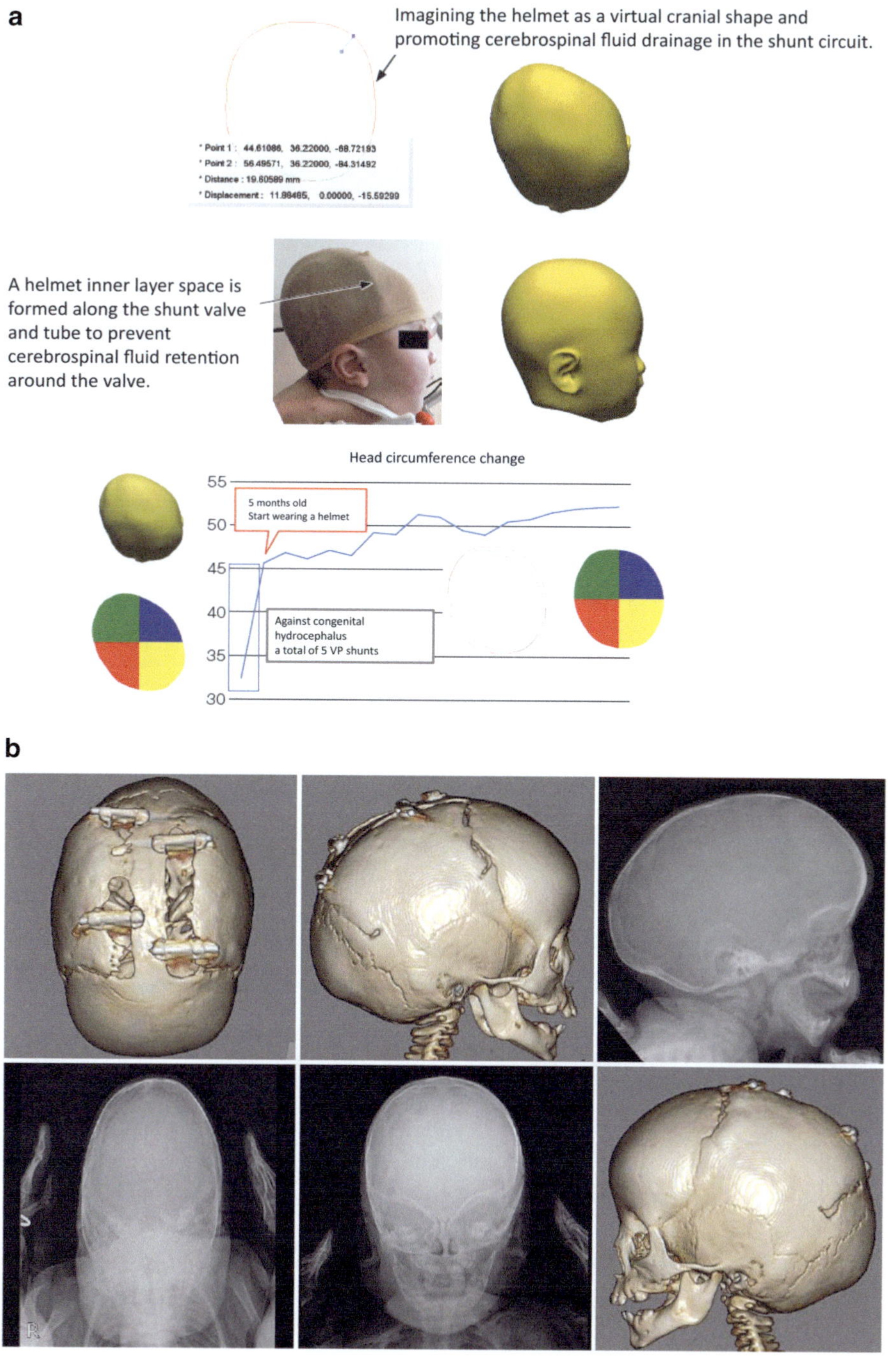

Fig. 15.2 (**a**) Cranial radiograph and 3D CT bone findings of premature cranial suture synostosis after surgical plastic surgery. (**b**) Corrective helmet wearing for premature cranial suture synostosis

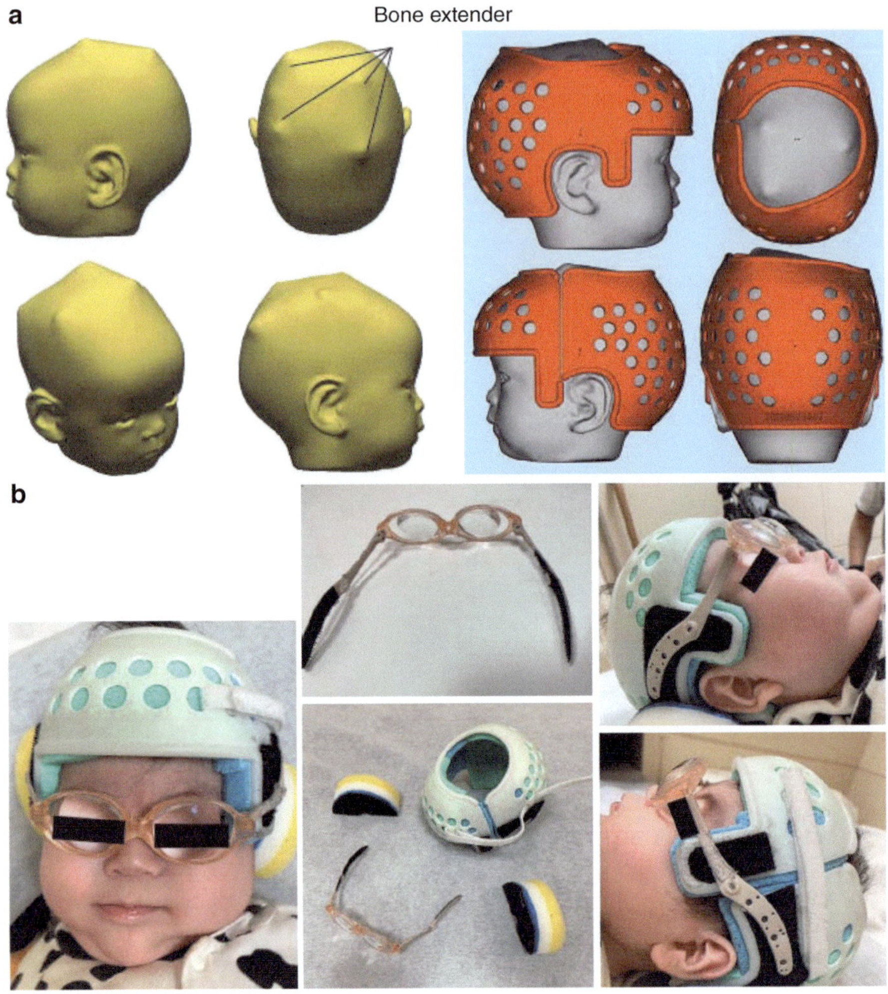

Fig. 15.3 Production of corrective glasses and orthotic helmets for retinopathy of prematurity. (©Nabeco)

according to the shape, but air leaks occur if the mask is not compressed to some extent, so the band fixing pressure is inevitably high.

With the Aimet®, by adding some ingenuity to the shape of the inner and outer layers of the helmet, it is possible to safely perform cranial orthotic treatment simultaneously, even for children who need to wear a CPAP mask for some time (Fig. 15.4).

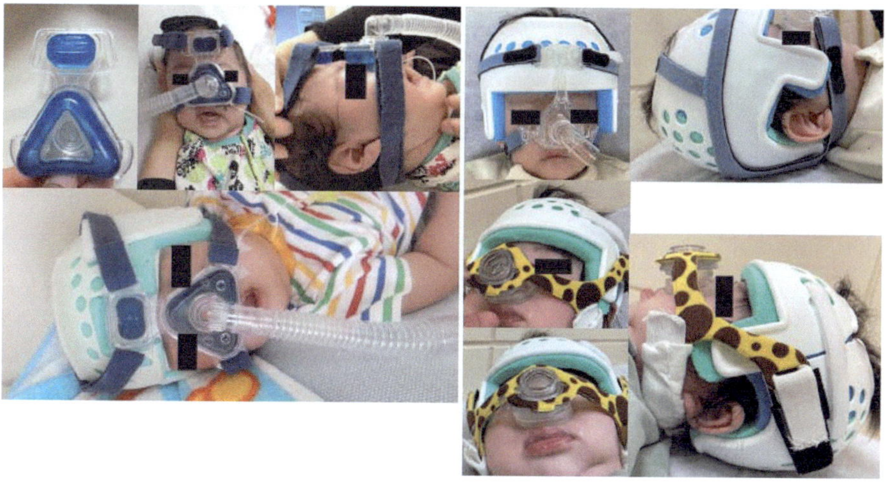

Fig. 15.4 Attaching an orthotic helmet to a child who needs a continuous positive airway pressure (CPAP) mask. (©Nabeco)

5 Torticollis and Hip Dislocation

Rehabilitation treatment for infant torticollis is often difficult. Orthotic helmet treatment can be expected not only to correct the cranial shape but also to assist in torticollis and conversion of the trunk to the contralateral side. In addition, it has been pointed out that cranial deformity progresses during the period of postural fixation due to wearing Remenbugel Hip Dislocation Brace. Even in patients who are older and generally considered difficult to undergo cranial orthotic treatment, there is a high possibility that orthotic effects can be expected if the patency of the anterior fontanelle is high. Sufficient consideration is required.

Chapter 16
Issues and Prospects of Orthotic Helmet Treatment

Yasuo Aihara

1 Correction Mechanism and Its Effect

Skull orthotic treatment with an orthotic helmet does not correct the skull by applying positive pressure to tighten the deformed skull with padding. The corrective mechanism is to delay the growth of the deformed skull in the longitudinal direction and promote the growth of the skull on the plagiocephaly side without hindering the expansion of the head circumference of normal infants. At that time, it is important for a skilled doctor to set and design the inner layer structure of the orthotic helmet according to the growth of the infant's skull, and to further adjust it according to the growth of the child.

It is possible to obtain a sufficient correction effect safely if it is started at 2–6 months after birth. The following three points show the effect of helmet correction treatment in Japan so far:

1. The sooner the treatment is started, the higher the corrective effect is, and it is highest especially in children before 4 months of age.
2. Corrective effect can be obtained if treatment is started before 6 months of age.
3. The earlier the age at which treatment is initiated, the higher the average post-treatment cranial symmetry ratio, and the correction effect is significantly lower when treatment is initiated at 9 months or older [1].

Y. Aihara (✉)
Department of Neurosurgery, Tokyo Women's Medical University, Tokyo, Japan
e-mail: yaihara@twmu.ac.jp

S. Kusuda et al. (eds.), *Handbook of Positional Plagiocephaly*,
https://doi.org/10.1007/978-981-97-9164-4_16

2 What Is the True Purpose of Treatment for Cranial Deformity?

What is the purpose of orthotic helmet treatment for positional cranial deformities in infancy? In actual clinical practice, there are many cases in which the parents of the affected children themselves have suffered from trunk balance disorders caused by severe cranial deformity, and so they wish to have their children corrected for the prevention of the disadvantage suffered. In severe positional plagiocephaly, not only is the complication rate of ipsilateral temporomandibular joint displacement (temporomandibular joint disorder) high, but ipsilateral torticollis is also frequently associated. The frequency of occlusion disorders, headaches, and stiff shoulders increases. Furthermore, to correct the collapsed trunk balance, there is a tendency for the shoulder position on the opposite side of plagiocephaly to drop. As a result, school-age children cannot carry school bags or rucksacks straight on their backs, causing slippage and the shoulder straps digging into their necks. Linked to the displacement of the shoulder position, there is a high tendency for scoliosis on the opposite side to compensate for trunk balance from the lowered shoulder position, which ultimately leads to complaints of low back pain and hip joint pain from pelvic displacement. This state is considered to be a phenomenon similar to the pathological condition in which the collapsed trunk balance due to positional plagiocephaly is compensated for by torticollis and elevated scapulae.

This should be recognized as an issue that affects future health and quality of life, rather than just cosmetic issues.

3 Interdisciplinary Cooperation Among Specialized Fields

Due to the lack of data on the average skull shape of infants in the East Asian regions, it is necessary to establish a classification of plagiocephaly deformity to establish helmet correction treatment for cranial deformity in Japan in the future. In addition to judging the suitability of orthotic helmet treatment, the establishment of universal cranial medical examinations, diagnosis, and treatment methods requires many health professionals, including perinatal care specialists (obstetricians, neonatologists, midwives, and nurses), pediatricians, rehabilitation specialists, orthopedic surgeons, plastic surgeons, otolaryngologists, dental and oral surgeons, and neurosurgeons.

Furthermore, to share the importance of cranial deformity prevention among health professionals, it is necessary to consider adding "diagnostic items for cranial deformity" to the *Maternal and Child Health Handbook* in the future.

Reference

1. Aihara Y, Chiba K, Kawamata T. Helmet therapy efficacy and its prediction in Japanese infants with positional plagio- and brachycephaly. Childs Nerv Syst. 2024.

Part IV
Questions and Answers

Chapter 17
Question and Answer (Q&A) for Cranial Deformity

Shigeharu Hosono

1 Basic Questions About Distortions of the Head

Q. Will the distortion of the head heal naturally?

If the distortion is mild, it will disappear as the baby grows, but if the distortion progresses to a moderate or higher level as the baby ages, it will be difficult to improve naturally.
At 1–2 months old, you can prevent the progression of distortion by paying attention to the direction of the head and laying it down.

Q. Can I change the orientation?

A. It is possible to consciously turn the baby upside down until around 1–2 months old, but it is difficult after that. Many babies have a preferred orientation from the time they are in their mother's womb. It's a baby's preference, so it can be said that it is very difficult to force a change.
Those who are born without orientation habits do not develop them during the first 1–2 weeks of life.

Q. Is the distortion caused by the lack of care for the baby?
Is it the mother's fault?

A. The way a child is raised does not determine their orientation. Just like there is a dominant hand, the baby's favorite direction is naturally determined. In some cases, the deformation has already started during pregnancy.

Q. If I change the child's posture (or if they start rolling over), will the distortion of the head naturally go away?

S. Hosono (✉)
Saitama Medical Center, Jichi Medical University, Saitama, Japan
e-mail: hosono.s@jichi.ac.jp

S. Kusuda et al. (eds.), *Handbook of Positional Plagiocephaly*,
https://doi.org/10.1007/978-981-97-9164-4_17

A. If the degree of distortion is mild, it may be improved to the extent that it is not noticeable. It is not realistic to return the head position each time when the baby is able to move the neck on its own after 2 months of age.
In addition, by laying the patient in the opposite direction, the pressure on the facing side will be dispersed, but it will not be a treatment to promote the growth of the original facing part and to promote the growth of other parts in a well-balanced manner. Hence, until you can sit down, it may remain as it is or may be deformed.

Q. Does head tilt due to torticollis require treatment?

A. Torticollis treatment may be required to prevent subsequent complications. If you are concerned about the shape of your baby's head, we recommend that you consult a specialized medical institution as soon as possible.
Torticollis is a condition in which the head is always tilted to one side or the other. Since the orientation of the face tends to be biased in one direction, it may have the same effect as the orientation. Torticollis can be caused by several factors, so the first thing to do is talk to your pediatrician or orthopedic surgeon.

Q. I'm worried that my child's head circumference is too big and that it's out of the growth curve.

A. Please plot the measured values from birth on the head circumference growth curve in the *Maternal and Child Health Handbook.*
If it is above the normal range, or if it is growing rapidly and approaching the upper limit of normal, please consult your pediatrician first.

Q. How long will the head shape continue to grow?

A. While there are individual differences, as you can see from the head circumference growth curve in the *Maternal and Child Health Handbook*, the baby's skull grows rapidly by about 7 months after birth and continues to grow thereafter. After 1 year of age, growth slows down, and by around one and a half years of age, the shape is almost fixed.

Q. Looking at the growth curve of the head circumference, it seems that growth slows down with age.

A. A baby's head circumference expands rapidly by about 7 months of age as the brain grows. From there, it will grow slowly. In addition, there are individual differences, so it cannot be said unconditionally, but from about 7 months after the growth becomes gentle, the treatment period will be longer with orthotic helmet treatment, and the treatment effect will be greater than those who started before 7 months.

Q. Is this distortion of the head hereditary?

A. While it is rare, there is a genetic abnormality that distorts the head, so in such cases, it may be inherited.

Orientation distortion is common. Even if it is not a hereditary disease, in rare cases, it may be distorted due to torticollis, so if you are concerned, please consult a pediatrician.

Q. It seems that the head is bumpy.

A. When a baby is born, the bones of its head (skull) have not yet joined together and are divided into several separate pieces. Shortly after birth, it is natural to have some unevenness because of childbirth and the joints of bones after birth. Please consult at your health checkup or visit a pediatrician if you are concerned.

Q. What is dolichocephaly?

A. When the head is longer than its width.

Q. What is brachycephaly?

A. It refers to the state in which the front–back diameter of the head is shorter than the width. It is medically distinguished from occipital flattening in which the roundness of the occipital region has disappeared. The brachycephaly may also be accompanied by the occipital deformity. Occipital flattening is commonly called precipice head.

Q. What is plagiocephaly?

A. A condition in which one side of the skull is obliquely distorted. There are frontal and occipital distortions. Angular plagiocephaly commonly occurs at the back of the head.

Q. What is crown tension?

A. The crown is a line that wraps around the head and refers to the part of the head that protrudes the most. When the tension of this part is large, it is called bee tension.

Q. What is premature cranial suture synostosis?

A. The skull is made up of bones such as the frontal, temporal, parietal, and occipital bones, and these bones fuse together more quickly than usual. At birth, the bones are not completely joined together, and as they grow, the bones become hard and fuse together. If this fusion occurs faster than normal, the bone cannot grow. The distorted shape of the head is caused by the difference in bone growth between areas where the skull is fused and where it is not. Surgery is generally required.

Q. I have plagiocephaly. Is it a disease?

A. Plagiocephaly occurs as a physiological phenomenon in infants who sleep on their backs. In rare cases, plagiocephaly is caused by an underlying disease; but in most cases, it is due to non-pathological factors such as turning. Treatment may be required depending on the degree of distortion. It is difficult to determine whether plagiocephaly is caused by an illness, so if you are concerned about the distortion, please consult a pediatrician.

Q. What is positional cranial deformity?

A. Positional cranial deformity is a distortion of the baby's head caused by external forces such as the effects of delivery, e.g., suction delivery, or the orientation of the head during sleep after birth.

Q. I'm worried that the image of trigonocephaly that I searched on the net and the shape of my child's head are similar.

A. First, please consult your family doctor. If a pathological condition is suspected, an X-ray examination or a CT examination will be performed at a specialized medical institution.

2 Questions about the Guideline for Consultation

Q. My family pediatrician says, "There is no need for any particular treatment," but is that okay?

A. Distortion of the head is not described in the Japanese pediatric textbooks, and there is no guidance for diagnosis and treatment. Some medical institutions have specialized outpatient clinics, so if you have any questions, please visit them.

Q. Is it okay to wait until about a few months after birth?

A. There are large individual differences, but in general, we recommend that you see a specialized medical institution as soon as possible, around the age of 6 months. In addition to treatment decisions, you can also receive advice such as preventive measures.

Q. When should I see a specialist?

A. If your family is worried about distortion, please consult a specialized medical institution. Appropriate advice will be given depending on the identification and degree of the cause of the distortion. Orthotic helmet treatment begins between the ages of 3 and 6 months and has the highest rate of improvement.

Q. Is it necessary to perform helmet correction treatment for the distortion of the baby's head?

A. Orthotic helmet treatment is not a prerequisite for consultation. At the first visit, the degree of distortion is checked by visual inspection and palpation. If there is distortion, determine if the distortion is provoked by pathological causes. Depending on the age of the patient and the degree of distortion, many

people receive lifestyle guidance and undergo follow-up observation, or, do not need to see a doctor after that.
In addition, even if it is diagnosed as severe, helmet correction treatment is not necessarily a treatment that must be performed, so please consider it after listening to the doctor's explanation.

Q. How much distortion should I consider helmet correction treatment?

A. Orthotic helmet treatment is performed when there is moderate or more distortion, such as the front and back positions of both ears being misaligned. Regardless of orthotic helmet treatment, informed consent (agreeing to a sufficient explanation from the doctor) is the basis for diagnosis and treatment, so please consult well.

Q. I feel that my ears are out of place. Should I see a doctor?

A. If the ear position is shifted forward or backward, the distortion may be moderate or higher. The degree of distortion can be determined by inspection and palpation by an experienced physician.

Q. I found a site called "Baby Head Shape Counseling Room" on the net. What is it for?

A. It was in the 1990s that the shape of the head began to be viewed as a potential problem. Plagiocephaly increased after the advocacy of avoiding sleeping on one's stomach and sleeping on one's back until the patient was able to turn over to prevent sudden infant death syndrome (SIDS). In the United States, the disease concept of positional plagiocephaly has now been established, but in our country, there is no medical education program regarding the prevention and treatment of this disease, so even pediatricians are in the minority who can provide correct information.
This site was initiated by a medical device manufacturer to provide reliable information on head distortions in babies, in collaboration with physicians who are well versed in positional plagiocephaly, and to indicate appropriate treatment initiation times and options. This is a consultation desk.
If necessary, we will help you find a hospital, and we aim to reduce the number of cases where effective treatment is overdue even if there is a possibility that you may be eligible for treatment.

3 Questions for Your First Visit

Q. Do I need a letter of introduction?

A. University hospitals and general hospitals that have a selected medical care system require a referral letter. If you do not have a letter of introduction, some hospitals allow you to see a doctor if you pay the selected medical expenses. You can visit the clinic without a letter of introduction.

Q. I cannot get a referral letter from my family pediatrician.

A. Some doctors decide that they don't need a referral letter even if they tell them they want it. In that case, please consult with another doctor or visit a specialized medical institution after paying the selected medical expenses. The clinic does not require a letter of introduction. A referral letter issued by a non-pediatrician or dentist is also acceptable.

Q. Please tell me about the selected medical expenses.

A. This is the cost for the first visit to a hospital with more than 200 beds without a letter of introduction. No re-examination is required. The amount varies depending on the hospital, but in many cases, it is around 5000–8000 yen. Even if you do not have a letter of introduction, you may be able to see a doctor by paying the selected medical expenses, so please inquire at the hospital.

Q. I have heard that it is difficult to make an appointment for a specialized outpatient clinic.

A. The number of medical institutions nationwide that have specialist outpatient clinics for head shape remains small, and some medical institutions require appointments 1–2 months in advance. First, contact the medical institution of your choice to check the reservation status.

Q. I am worried about radiation exposure from an X-ray examination of the head.

A. There is no need to worry as the radiation dose will be adjusted for the baby. Although the amount of radiation exposure from a single imaging session is small compared to the natural radiation exposure you receive in your normal life, please consult your doctor before imaging.

Q. Does scanning affect the human body?

A. It is the same as taking a picture with a smartphone camera, so there is no effect on the human body.

Q. How long is the valid period of scanned data?

A. It depends on the facility, but most of them say within a week at the longest. Because the shape of the baby's head changes day by day. We manufacture helmets based on scanned data and provide helmets that are designed to be effective approximately 2 weeks after ordering. If the data becomes old, the shape of the head will change during this period, which will hinder effective helmet production.

Q. How is distortion diagnosed? Is it digitized?

A. It is common to synthesize the results of scanning with the camera in three dimensions, digitize the measured values, and classify them as mild, moderate, severe, and extremely severe.

Q. Which department should I consult at the hospital?
Are you a pediatrician? Are you a neurosurgeon? Is it plastic surgery?

A. Many of the medical institutions that have outpatient clinics specializing in head shape require a referral letter, so please consult your pediatrician first.

Q. Can I consult with the head shape outpatient clinic even if my head is slightly distorted?

A. Head shape outpatient clinic is not an outpatient clinic for helmet correction treatment. It is an outpatient clinic where you can receive consultations, including the introduction of preventive methods, for families of babies who are concerned about the shape of their heads. Positional plagiocephaly is not the only cause of head deformity, so we will consider prevention and treatment after conducting a differential diagnosis. Please feel free to contact us.

4 Questions About Home Care and Other Treatments

Q. How can I change my orientation?

A. It's a baby's preference, so it's difficult to change. In addition, if the head is distorted, the baby will naturally face the better side of the head. However, they will sleep with the side that is distorted down. This becomes a habit and it will further encourage the distortion of the baby's head.

Q. What can you do at home to deal with your baby's head distortion?

A. Traditionally, there are corrective pillows (doughnut pillows), calling from the opposite side of the person's facing direction (adjusting the bed to the direction the family is), putting a towel on the back and fixing it, and turning the patient frequently. There is such care. However, as the baby gets older, they will start to move their neck on their own, so there are limits to this type of care. In addition, be careful when using towels and pillows as they pose a choking hazard. One way to breastfeed is to face the opposite side of the direction you often face.
It is important to devise ways not to take a fixed position as much as possible.

Q. What is Tummy Time?

A. A tummy is a child's word "pom-pon", which means "tummy." In Japan, it is said to be "lie down practice (play)" or "belly practice (play)." Lie face down on your mother's or father's body (sometimes on a hard floor or mat) 2–4 times a day for 5 min at first, and then for a total of 20 min once you get

used to it. For babies who have been sleeping on their backs for a long time, putting them on their stomachs is said to be good for preventing head distortion and for developing muscles in the upper body, such as the neck.
Placing an infant on its stomach to sleep is strictly prohibited as it is a risk factor for SIDS. Always do it when the baby is awake, and the parents will also be able to do it without hesitation by lying on their stomachs and making eye contact. Rather than correcting the distortion, these are done to prevent the distortion from slowing down the progression or not causing the distortion.

Q. Is the bodywork effective?

A. There is a chiropractic clinic in Japan that claims that it can be effective for plagiocephaly, but medical evidence is insufficient. Some places recommend a combination with orthotic helmet treatment, but this is also not a sufficient medical basis.
Although it is different from manipulative treatment if you have plagiocephaly due to torticollis, the opening of the hip joint on the opposite side to which your face is facing may be poor, so in that case, physical therapy may be performed.

5 Questions About Effects of Cranial Deformity

Q. I heard that the Ministry of Health, Labor, and Welfare has published a report on the effects on development.

A. The Japanese Society of Plastic and Reconstructive Surgery has requested a shape-guided helmet, and in response to this, it is the material reported at the 22nd Study Group on Early Introduction of Medical Devices with High Medical Needs. It can be viewed on the website of the Ministry of Health, Labor, and Welfare.
[https://www.mhlw.go.jp/file/05-Shingikai-11121000-Iyakushokuhinkyoku-Soumuka/0000055706_4.pdf]
Among them, "Cranial deformation due to external pressure in infancy has been thought not to cause growth and developmental delay or functional impairment", but cases with deformative plagiocephaly may affect neurodevelopment and motor development. There are multiple reports that it is accompanied by delay. In cases such as those associated with muscular torticollis that does not respond to positive posture changes for a certain time, or in cases where a high degree of orientation is maintained, the cranial deformity may spontaneously improve. From the perspective of preventing delays in neurodevelopment and motor development, it is considered that treatment is positively indicated for moderate to severe degenerative plagiocephaly.

Q. What are the dangers of not getting treatment?

A. The exact frequency is unknown, but domestic and international papers have reported delays in motor and neurodevelopment. In clinical practice, it has been pointed out that facial asymmetry affects jaw distortion, scoliosis, strabismus, stiff shoulders, migraines, and tooth alignment. In addition, it is said that there is a risk that it will lead to difficulty in wearing glasses.

Q. Is it true that there is also an intellectual delay?

A. There is no need to worry too much unless the head is distorted due to illness. Please consult your pediatrician if you have any concerns about the shape of the head.

Q. Will it affect the alignment of my teeth?

A. There are reports that it affects the alignment of the teeth, but the causal relationship is not clear.

Q. Is there a risk of strabismus?

A. It has been reported that people with plagiocephaly often have strabismus. A study published in 2007 by Professor Ricci et al. of the Catholic University of Italy on the evaluation of visual function in infants associated with head deformity reported a high prevalence of strabismus and asymmetric visual field in children with plagiocephaly.1) Of the infants presenting with head flattening, 84% had some form of visual dysfunction, 55% of which had oculomotor abnormalities, including strabismus, and 45% had visual field abnormalities. In addition to visual dysfunction, these children have been shown to have a high prevalence of headaches.
A squint may be the cause of torticollis. If you are concerned about strabismus, see an ophthalmologist.

6 Questions About Orthotic Helmet Treatment

Timing of Indication and Initiation of Treatment

Q. In what cases is orthotic helmet treatment possible?

A. This is possible when the head is distorted due to deformation or orientation due to childbirth. Treatment is given under the supervision of a doctor. If there is a distortion in the head due to some disease, treatment of the causal disease is necessary.

Q. When is the right age to start orthotic helmet treatment?

A. It is said to be 3–6 months after birth, but the timing of starting helmet correction treatment is determined comprehensively based on the severity of the head distortion at the time of the first visit and the progress of the distortion during follow-up. After the appropriate age, it becomes difficult to improve the distortion. If you are concerned about distortion, please consult a specialized medical institution as soon as possible.

Q. I would like to receive treatment as soon as possible. At what age can I start treatment?

A. If the distortion is large, it may start about 2 months after birth.

Q. I have a question regarding Down Syndrome. Can I get orthotic helmet treatment?

A. Since children with Down syndrome grow slowly, such as turning over and acquiring a sitting position, there is currently little information on the duration and efficacy of treatment. Since Down syndrome varies greatly from person to person, first please consult your pediatrician.

Q. Is it effective even if it is distorted due to suction delivery or forceps delivery?

A. Therapeutic effect can be expected.

Q. Is it effective for deformation due to cephalohematoma?

A. Cephalohematoma itself is naturally resorbed, but if it is caused by cephalohematoma and causes distortion, treatment may be indicated, so please consult a doctor as soon as possible.

Q. Cephalic hematomas are present on the left and right sides and are hard and calcified. The head is flat when viewed from the front, and the shape of the face is like a home base. Is it better to remove the calcified material before the orthotic helmet treatment, or can it be done without removing it?

A. If you have a head hematoma, you may have a head tilt as a result. If you are concerned, please consult a specialized medical institution. Even if you have cephalohematoma, orthotic helmet treatment may be possible.

Q. Can you make a diagnosis by looking at the photos taken with the measurement app?

A. The app is intended to be used as a guide only. At a specialized medical institution, the shape of the child's head is inspected and palpated, and the child's age is considered before deciding whether to follow up or undergo helmet correction treatment.

6.1 Treatment Know-How

Q. What is the general flow of treatment?

A. At the first visit, we will investigate the cause of the distortion of the head. If the cause is external pressure such as the effects of childbirth or misalignment, a special device is used to measure the degree of distortion. Depending

on the age and degree of distortion, we will determine whether helmet correction treatment is required.
If it is considered that orthotic helmet treatment is required, we will explain the treatment period, visit intervals, effects, complications, costs, and so on to the family again. If you wish to have orthotic helmet treatment, we will create a helmet suitable for the child based on the scan data.

Q. How long does it take to make a helmet?

A. After a 3D scan, it takes approximately 2 weeks to make the helmet. Since the shape and size of the child's head change day by day, it is made considering that.

Q. How often will I have to visit the doctor once treatment has started?

A. To change the cushion inside the helmet according to the degree of growth of the head, you will have to go to the outpatient clinic about once a month. For a standard 6-month treatment period, the number of consultations is six times and for a longer treatment period of 12 months it is 12 times.

Q. How long is the treatment period?

A. Although it depends on the severity of the strain and the growth of the head, 6 months is standard, and in some cases, it is longer than 12 months.

Q. Please tell me the goal of the wearing time per day.

A. The target for wearing time per day is 23 h. However, instead of wearing it for a long time from the first day of correction, gradually increase the time over approximately 2 weeks. For example, Day 1: 4 h, Day 2: 5 h, Day 5: 12 h, and so on. The corrective effect can be particularly expected at bedtime (when the head is on the ground).

Q. What is the frequency of 3D scanning?
Will I have a scan every time I see a doctor?

A. 3D scanning is always performed when making a cranial correction helmet, but the interval between subsequent 3D scanning varies depending on the degree of improvement in the deformation rate due to medical examination and the way of thinking of each medical institution. The general policy will be explained by the doctor in charge when starting the helmet correction treatment.

Q. Is it possible to make a second helmet?

A. Generally, it can be treated with one helmet. There is rarely a need to craft a second helmet.

Q. I don't understand the difference between a 3D scanner and a 3D printer.

A. A scanner is to take pictures to acquire data. A 3D printer is a machine that creates 3D objects based on that data.

Q. I am undergoing orthotic helmet treatment, can I change hospitals?

A. Orthotic helmet treatment is a free practice, so we accept patients and secure reservation slots on the premise that they will continue to receive treatment until the end of treatment at the facility where the helmet was ordered. Since it is not a treatment that is performed anywhere in Japan, there are currently few hospitals that accept transfer patients. In addition, even if you find a place to accept it, you will have to bear new costs such as remaking the helmet.

Q. Does the ideal head shape differ depending on the doctor's idea?

A. The goal is to have a round head with less left and right asymmetry. Therefore, the head is photographed from multiple directions to create a 3D image of the head, and the helmet is made accordingly, so the doctor's subjectivity is not included.

6.2 Questions, Anxieties, and Concerns About Treatment

Q. I am worried that the orthotic helmet treatment will put stress on my baby.

A. It is medically and objectively difficult to judge whether orthotic helmet treatment is stressful for babies. Orthotic helmet treatment is painless when done properly. There are also consultations such that it became difficult to turn over and wake up at night. Many babies adapt.

Q. My grandparents are against orthotic helmet treatment.
Do you have any advice?

A. If the patient has objected before undergoing a medical examination, explain that the distortion of the head may be caused by an underlying disease such as premature cranial suture synostosis, go to the outpatient clinic together, and receive an explanation from the doctor.
If you are opposed to the cost, you may be able to get medical expense assistance, so I will explain that as well.

Q. I live in an area where it is very cold in winter. Is there any problem with orthotic helmet treatment?

A. The temperature environment does not interfere with treatment.

Q. Will babies wear helmets properly? Isn't it possible to remove it yourself?

A. Some babies don't like it because of the start time and individual differences, but many of those babies adapt. If you start at an advanced age, you may take it off by yourself when you are about 1 year old, but in that case, you can continue treatment by devising things such as wearing a helmet after you sleep.

Q. Are there any side effects?

A. There are reports of skin troubles such as heat rash and rashes. If you have a skin problem, we will recommend treatment while consulting with a dermatologist.

Q. Are there any concerns that the treatment may delay development?

A. Orthotic helmet treatment slows down the growth of the protruding part and creates space in the part that has become flat due to pressure to promote the original growth. It does not tighten the head to correct it. There have been no reports that orthotic helmet treatment causes some kind of brain disorder and delays development.

Q. Why is the top of the helmet open?
If I have a long head, can I correct the top of the head?

A. Brachycephaly refers to cases in which the head is not vertically long when viewed from the front but is long in the front–back direction when viewed from the top (parietal side). Helmets are not designed to correct long crown-to-chin shapes.
The reason for the hole in the top of the head is the structural problem that the helmet cannot be opened, the fact that even if the top of the head is blocked, there is no effect of suppressing the target area, and the weight reduction and good ventilation are ensured.

Q. What materials are the helmet and cushions made of?

A. The shell part is made of a special nylon resin. The cushion is made of soft urethane foam, a type of low-resilience material. This material has less localized pressure and spreads the pressure on the head all over, so it has the effect of blocking blood flow and preventing chafing, making it gentle on babies' fragile skin. It also has some amount of shock absorption. It is also used for pillows, futons, and mattresses.

Q. If you must give up treatment in the middle, in what cases?

A. In addition to some circumstances on the family side, there are cases where the child develops an ego and begins to remove the helmet, and the treatment may be terminated.

Q. I would like to receive treatment, but there are only hospitals far from my home. Is telemedicine treatment possible? What method do you use?

A. Some medical institutions have introduced telemedicine, but face-to-face medical care is required for the first visit, the first time wearing a helmet, and the decision to end the treatment. It is up to the medical institution to decide how many times during the 6–12-month treatment period to use telemedicine.

Examining while sharing images with a camera and interacting remotely is a method of telemedicine. The cushioning material for the helmet will be sent separately, so the family will have to reupholster the cushion under the direction of the doctor.

6.3 *About the Effects of Treatment*

Q. Is it not possible to expect the effect if the age is progressing?

A. It is more effective to wear a helmet when the growth of the head is remarkable. Therefore, it is effective to start treatment before the age of 3–6 months. However, there are individual differences in growth, so please consult a doctor as soon as possible.

Q. Will the misaligned ears be cured with orthotic helmet treatment?

A. As plagiocephaly becomes more severe, the sunken side of the ear shifts forward. As plagiocephaly improves, it is expected that the ear position will return to its original position.

Q. Is there a rebound?

A. There is no rebound in the etiology of positional plagiocephaly.

6.4 *About the Cost of Treatment*

Q. Is orthotic helmet treatment covered by insurance?

A. Diagnosis of the cause of head distortion and follow-up without making a helmet are covered by insurance. Making a helmet, then visiting an outpatient clinic about once a month, and adjusting the cushion inside the helmet are free medical treatments. In the case of clinics, all medical care may be free.

Q. Is the first visit covered by insurance?

A. At general medical institutions, the first visit is usually covered by health insurance. Some clinics that specialize in the shape of the head offer free medical care. Many of them are listed on the websites of medical institutions, so please check in advance. In addition, it is important to double-check when booking.

Q. Is there any assistance for financial burdens such as final tax returns?

A. It is eligible for medical expense deduction. Please let us know when you file your tax return. Ultimately, it will be decided by the tax office, but basically, the refund will be based on the annual household income. In addition, please consider applying to the health insurance association, for the cost of medical equipment as medical expenses. However, it is up to the association to decide whether they are eligible, and it seems that in many cases they are not accepted.

6.5 *Precautions During Treatment*

Q. The helmet comes off easily, what should I do?

A. The shell of the helmet is custom-made to suit the individual. We expect to be able to use it until the end of treatment with a single fabrication, so we set a space between the head shape and the shell that does not hinder growth so that the ideal head shape will be achieved at the end of treatment. In addition, the shell alone will rotate or come off, so use a sponge with an appropriate thickness to fill the gap. While maintaining the necessary space until the next medical examination for correction, the thickness of the sponge is adjusted so that it does not come off frequently.
In rare cases, when treatment is started early or in severely ill children, even if the fit is confirmed during the initial adjustment, it may come off easily after use. If you feel that it is easy to take off after wearing it for the first time, please consult a doctor as soon as possible.

Q. Can I wear a knit hat when wearing a helmet?

A. There are reports of skin problems such as heat rashes and rashes caused by wearing a helmet. The large holes in the top of the helmet are for ventilation. If you put on a knit hat, this hole will be blocked, so the ventilation will not be maintained, and the temperature inside the helmet will rise and become stuffy, causing skin problems.
Moreover, at this age, I don't think he goes out on rainy days very often, but even when putting on a hooded raincoat, if you put a hood on your head, heat may get trapped inside the helmet, so be careful.

Q. Is it possible to accept children at the nursery school during orthotic helmet treatment?

A. Please check first with the nursery school you wish to enter. The Basic Act on Childrearing, which came into force on December 1, 2019, includes enhancements to support systems for children requiring medical care and caregivers.
Nursery schools that have no experience accepting such children may be hesitant to accept children because they think they need something special. Parents can use a pamphlet to provide a detailed explanation or submit a medical certificate from the doctor in charge to help them understand. If the child is

still not accepted, why not ask the kindergarten doctor to check with the nursery school?

6.6 Maintenance of Orthotic Helmet

Q. If the inside of the helmet gets wet with sweat, is it okay to dry it with a hair dryer?

A. If it gets wet with sweat, do not remove the cushion from the shell and dry it with cool air from the inside. Avoid drying with a hot air dryer as it will damage the cushion.

Q. Can the cushion be washed with water?

A. Cushion cannot be washed with water. If you are concerned, please use a product (nonalcoholic disinfectant spray "Interception" Fuji Techno Service Co., Ltd.) that has been confirmed to have no problems by verifying compatibility with the material.

Q. Can the helmet be washed with water?

A. The shell part of the helmet can be washed with water, but it will soak into the inside and the cushion will get wet, so if the dirt is noticeable, wipe the outside of the shell with water. If the cushion gets wet, it will become stuffy, so remove the cushion from the shell and let it dry.

Q. Will the white color of the helmet fade or transfer?

A. The white color of the helmet is the color of the nylon resin material, so the color will not fade or transfer.

Q. Can I care for the cushions at home?

A. There is no need for any special techniques or tools, so if you receive proper instructions on how to reupholster your cushions, you will be able to reupholster them easily at home. All you have to do is peel off the existing cushion, cut out the new cushion material with the specified thickness using the paper pattern, and stick it in place (Fig. 17.1).

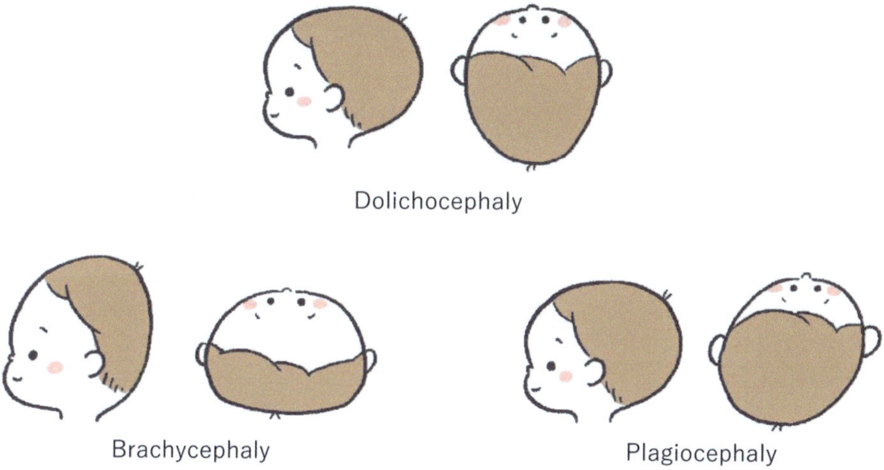

Fig. 17.1 Types of cranial deformation. (©Nabeco)

Reference

1. Ricci D, Vasco G, Baranello G, et al. Visual function in infants with non-syndromic craniosynostosis. Dev Med Child Neurol. 2007;49:574–6.

Glossary

1 Skull Deformities

Argenta's clinical classification In 2004, Argenta proposed a classification of the degree of cranial deformity based on inspection and palpation, which is classified into five stages from I to V. In clinical practice in Japan, I to IV are used (see Fig. 8). Argenta's paper does not describe the measured value of the front-to-back deviation of the left and right ears; however, in Japan, a displacement of 1 cm or more is considered abnormal.

Type I: Cranial asymmetry is limited to the occiput, with varying degrees of occipital flattening. No anteroposterior asymmetry is noted between the left and right ears, and the face is bilaterally symmetrical.

Type II: Cranial asymmetry is limited to the occiput, with varying degrees of occipital flattening. Severe cases are enough to displace the flat side of the ear forward, downward, or both. No facial asymmetry is observed.

Type III: This includes posterior skull asymmetry, ipsilateral ear malposition, and frontal asymmetry due to ipsilateral frontal protrusion but with preserved bilateral facial symmetry.

Type IV: This deformity is accompanied by occipital deformity, ipsilateral ear malposition, ipsilateral frontal asymmetry, and ipsilateral facial asymmetry.

Type V: In addition to type IV, bulging of the temporal region and abnormal vertical growth of the occipital region to avoid anatomical strain on the growing brain is observed.

Auricle position displacement The position of the auricles as seen from the front of the face is in a state in which there is a difference in height between the left and right sides of the line connecting the inner and outer can thus, or when viewed from the top of the head, the positions of the left and right auricles are shifted back and forth. As positional plagiocephaly increases in severity, the auricle on the plagiocephaly side is displaced forward.

S. Kusuda et al. (eds.), *Handbook of Positional Plagiocephaly*,
https://doi.org/10.1007/978-981-97-9164-4

Anterior fontanelle The anterior fontanelle is the area where the frontal, sagittal, right, and left coronal sutures of the skull meet. The area is a diamond-shaped bone gap and refers to the membranous tissue section. The anterior fontanelle is always present in the neonatal period, shrinks with growth, and closes at 12–18 months of age. Immediately after delivery, it may be difficult to recognize if there is an intussusception. However, individual differences in the timing of the closure of the anterior fontanelle are large, and even in healthy children, it may already be closed 3 to 4 months after birth; thus, a diagnosis by a specialist is recommended.

Brachycephaly This condition occurs when the cephalic index, which is the percentage of head width to head length, is 81% or more. Brachycephaly should be distinguished from occipital flattening, which is a condition in which the occipital region is flattened due to an increased radius of curvature of the occipital region, although it may coexist. Occipital flattening is commonly referred to as precipice head.

Compensatory enlargement of head circumference This enlargement is recognized as a symptom of increased intracranial pressure in infants. In infancy, the skull is not fused; thus, even if intracranial pressure is increased, suture separation occurs, compensating for the increase of intracranial pressure and causing head circumference enlargement.

Cranial asymmetry (CA) CA is calculated using the following formula:

CA (mm) = diagonal line (B) − diagonal line A (B > A)

Note: The denominator (A) and numerator (B − A) are reversed in some reports.

Craniosynostosis The skulls of fetuses and newborns/infants are composed of multiple bones, and the gaps between them are called cranial sutures. As the infant grows, the skull bones gradually fuse. Craniosynostosis is a condition in which one or more of the cranial sutures fuses prematurely for any reason. As a result, the skull is deformed, and further growth of the head circumference is inhibited, resulting in microcephaly. In the glossary of the Japanese Association of Medical Sciences, the use of the term "*togaihogosokiyugosho*" is recommended; however, in the glossary of the Japan Pediatric Society, the terms "*togaikotsuyugosho*," "*togaikotsuhogosokiyugosho*," and "*togaihogosokikotsuka*" are also used.

Cranioplasty In craniosynostosis, surgery is performed to cut the deformed part of the skull and reassemble it into a shape close to a normal skull. At this time, a thread or plate that absorbs over time is used to fix the bones of the infant so as not to remain as a foreign substance as much as possible.

Cranial sutures The skull is made up of multiple bones, and during infancy, gaps are present between adjacent bones. This gap is called a suture line. Sutures appear black and linear on plain X-ray images of the head.

Cross-sectional growth chart of head circumference Cross-sectional growth chart of the head circumference is one of the physical growth curves for infants that is used to assess head circumference growth. The *Maternal and Child Health Handbook* also includes height and weight growth charts along with head circumference. Seven curves are drawn from the 3rd percentile to the 97th percentile, with the month and age on the horizontal axis and the head circumference on the vertical axis. The latest edition was created based on the 2010 Infant Physical Development Survey.

Dolichocephaly Dolichocephaly is a condition in which the cephalic index, which is the percentage of head width to head length, is 76% or more. The anteroposterior diameter of the head clearly increases compared with the lateral diameter. Although it should be distinguished from marked occipital protrusion due to reduced occipital radius of curvature, some of these cases may be complicated by dolichocephaly.

Enlarged head circumference Enlarged head circumference is an abnormal enlargement of the head circumference greater than age-matched mean + 2 standard deviations (SD) or greater than the 97th percentile of the head growth curve. Enlarged head circumference is also called macrocephaly. Furthermore, even if the head circumference is below the standard, caution should be exercised in expanding across the percentile curve in the short term.

Facial bone displacement Facial bone displacement is a condition in which craniosynostosis significantly inhibits growth not only of the head but also of the jaw and face three-dimensionally, resulting in facial asymmetry. In addition, facial asymmetry has also been reported in severe plagiocephaly.

Hachibari *Hachi* refers to the part of the parietal bone where a severe curvature of the head is present. This is called the *hachibari*, which refers to a part that is stretched. The part above the *hachi* (band) is called "band top," and the part below the band is called "band bottom." In general, it refers to the part around which a headband is wrapped.

Hydrocephalus The cerebrospinal fluid in the cranium (ventricle, subarachnoid space, etc.) accumulates excessively for some reason in this condition, causing the ventricle expansion. When cerebrospinal fluid accumulates mainly in the subarachnoid space on the brain surface, external hydrocephalus occurs.

Mandibular displacement Mandibular displacement is a condition in which the position of the mandible (jaw position) is slightly displaced from its normal position. As a result, the centers of the upper and lower teeth are misaligned, and the face becomes asymmetrical, making it difficult to chew food.

Meningitis Meningitis is a condition in which pathogens invade and infect the meninges that surround the brain, causing inflammation. The main causes of meningitis are bacteria, viruses, *Mycobacterium tuberculosis*, and fungi. In early infancy, symptoms, such as fever, vomiting, bulging fontanelle, and suture separation, occur.

Overlapping of cranial bones The skull of the fetus is incompletely ossified and soft, and bony sutures that are not yet fused between the sutures that make up the skull are present. Therefore, the head of the fetus can change its shape to some extent due to the pressure of the birth canal when passing through it. This deformation is called fetal head adaptation. In addition, each cranial bone can move and overlap with adjacent skulls, which is called overlapping of cranial bones. Cranial deformity due to overlapping of cranial bones improves within 2–3 days after birth and within 1 week at the latest.

Plagiocephaly Among skull deformities, plagiocephaly is a condition of left–right asymmetry of the skull. Causes are broadly classified into positional plagiocephaly, in which the contact surface of the head is deformed through external pressure in the uterus or the weight of the infant's own head after birth, and craniosynostosis caused by premature fusion of bone sutures. Among craniosynostosis, premature fusion of the unilateral coronal suture causes anterior plagiocephaly, and similarly, premature fusion of the unilateral lambdoid suture causes posterior plagiocephaly, which must be differentiated.

Positional skull deformity Cranial deformity is a general term for the condition in which the skull of an infant has deformed beyond a certain level, although cranial deformity has already occurred since the fetal period in some cases. Cranial deformity is caused by the influence of external pressure on the skull before birth, during delivery, and after birth, excluding skull deformity owing to pathological causes such as craniosynostosis. The deformity is also called nonsynostotic skull deformity because it does not involve cranial suture fusion. Cranial deformity is broadly classified into plagiocephaly, brachycephaly, and dolichocephaly; however, mixed types also exist.

Posterior fontanelle The posterior fontanelle is a triangular membranous tissue located between the parietal and occipital bones where the sagittal and humeral sutures meet. It closes before 6 months of age.

Positional plagiocephaly A condition where a baby's head develops a flat spot due to prolonged pressure on one area.

Cranial vault asymmetry index (CVAI)

CVAI is calculated using the following formula:

CVAI (%) = Diagonal (B) – Diagonal (A)/Diagonal (A) × 100 (B > A)

CVAI is the difference between the lengths of two diagonals 30°apart from the midline divided by the larger of the two diagonals. The higher the index, the more asymmetric the cranial vault is.

Note: The denominator (A) and numerator (B – A) are reversed in some reports.

Pathological cranial deformity Pathological cranial deformity is a condition caused by craniosynostosis. This condition is classified as nonsyndromic or symptomatic depending on the presence or absence of other comorbidities. Pathological cranial deformity does not improve with helmet orthodontic treatment alone, and surgical treatment is required for suture excision.

Surgical craniofacial reconstruction Surgical craniofacial reconstruction is the generic name for reconstructive surgery for craniofacial bone deformity through surgical procedures, with craniosynostosis (symptomatic and non-syndromic) as a representative disease. Conversely, cranial correction helmet treatment can be said to be a medical treatment method.

Symptoms of increased intracranial pressure This condition results from an increase in intracranial volume for some reason. Symptoms vary in infancy depending on the rate of increase in intracranial pressure. Acute intracranial pressure increase is associated with irritability, high-pitched crying, vomiting, lethargy, and bulging fontanelle. Suture dehiscence and widening of the head circumference are observed in chronic cases.

Trigonocephaly Trigonocephaly is a condition in which the skull is wedge-shaped or triangular when viewed from the parietal side. The top of the triangle is the mid front of the frontal area, and the base of the triangle is the occipital area.

2 Development

Asymmetrical tonic neck reflex (ATNR) ATNR is one of the primitive reflexes seen in newborns. When a newborn is laid on its back, and the face is turned to one side, the upper and lower limbs on the face side extend, and the occipital side bends. The reflex disappears after 4 months of age and is abnormal if it persists beyond 6 months of age.

Head control In general, head control is also called "*kubisuwari*" (holding up one's head) and refers to a state in which the neck does not wobble even if the back of the head is not supported. From a supine position, hold the child with both hands and slowly raise the child, pulling the chin at a 45° so that the head and trunk are aligned. If the head does not tilt forward when the head is raised to 90°, then the complete head control is recognized. Full-term infants usually have a head control by the age of 4 months, and the absence beyond 5 months is considered abnormal.

Rollover Rollover refers to going from a supine to a prone position, which is usually possible at 4–6 months of age. Rollover is sometimes distinguished from "re-rollover," which is a transition from prone to supine. However, the first timing of re-rollover is slightly later than that of rollover. In some cases, the period in which rolling over on only one side is possible lasts for a long time.

Smooth pursuit Eye movements occur in which an infant follows a moving object. Immediately after birth, newborns have poor visual acuity and poor smooth pursuit ability. As their eyesight gradually improves as they age, they can recognize objects 20–30 cm in front of them, and if they move slowly, they can follow them with their eyes. At 2 months of age, clear follow-up is observed along with fixation.

3 Risk of Plagiocephaly and Related Disorders

Dislocation of the hip The hip joint connects the pelvis and the lower limbs. Its shape allows the head of the femur to fit into the acetabulum (concave) on the pelvic side. This congenital misfit of the hip joint is called congenital hip dislocation. In Europe and the United States, the word "congenital" is not used and is called developmental dysplasia of the hip. The habit of facing the same direction often results in a kneeling position on the leg opposite the facing side, which can lead to hip dislocation.

Habit of facing the same direction This condition occurs when the face is always oriented toward the same direction when the newborn is placed in the supine position. In the womb, the fetus has already developed a habit of facing the same direction to some degree. If this condition continues, it may progress to plagiocephaly, in which the weight of the head flattens the skull on the ground.

Habit of facing the same direction (sleeping position) The habit is a consensus that "facing habit" refers to the position where newborns like to turn their head in one direction during sleeping. As long as no secondary factors, such as birth trauma, exist, this sleeping habit (facing habit) is said to be determined to some extent during the prenatal period. This habit is different from the commonly used meaning of "bed hair." This term is used in fields such as neurosurgery and plastic surgery.

Muscular torticollis This type of torticollis is caused by contraction of the sternocleidomastoid muscle that connects the back of the head to the clavicle/sternum. Typically, the neck is tilted to the affected side (the side that palpates the swollen muscle tissue (mass)), and the face is turned to the opposite side. The swollen muscle tissue reaches its maximum size at 2–3 weeks of age and then gradually shrinks spontaneously. Among cases of muscular torticollis, 80–90% heal spontaneously by the age of 18 months.

Secondary muscular torticollis Severe plagiocephaly may result in prolonged restricted neck rotation and a secondary increase in muscle tone in the sternocleidomastoid muscle on the opposite side of plagiocephaly. In such a condition, torticollis develops from plagiocephaly, and the restricted rotation due to torticollis continues to press on the plagiocephaly side, which may lead to a vicious cycle of aggravated plagiocephaly.

Strabismus Both eyes of the infant are directed toward the same place when gazing at an object. Strabismus is a condition in which the right and left eyes are looking in different directions. Strabismus is classified into esotropia, exotropia, up–down strabismus, rotator strabismus, and so on, according to the direction of deviation of the line of sight. Severe plagiocephaly with facial asymmetry may result in strabismus.

Traumatic muscular torticollis This type of torticollis is caused by a subluxation of the cervical vertebrae due to a strong force, or twisting force, applied to a specific part of the neck. In terms of age, onset is often in infancy. Subluxation is predominantly caused by atlantoaxial rotatory fixation (AARF) in which the atlas (first cervical vertebra) rotates forward while rotating with respect to the axis (second cervical vertebra).

Torticollis Torticollis is a condition in which the head and neck are always turned to one side or the other and cannot turn to the other side. The infants with this disorder are unable to face the front even when reacting. Muscular torticollis is the most common cause of torticollis in infancy. In addition, torticollis is classified as bony, inflammatory, and ocular. As infants with torticollis can only face in one direction, it causes positional plagiocephaly and plagiocephaly.

4 Related to Obstetrics

Cephalohematoma A lump that forms when the periosteum that covers the skull comes off due to pressure on the fetal head as it passes through the birth canal, and blood accumulates in the periosteum. It becomes more noticeable 2–3 days after birth rather than on the day of birth. It vibrates when touched and does not form a digital marking when pressed. Treatment is usually not required and is absorbed spontaneously in the first 2–3 months of life. Cephalohematomas do not extend beyond bony sutures. Caution should be exercised if the size of the cephalohematoma is large, as it may cause secondary cranial deformity (plagiocephaly).

Fetal position of presentation The orientation of the fetus in the uterus, expressed by the positional relationship between the uterus and the fetus in the longitudinal direction, is classified into head, breech, and lateral positions. The part of the fetal body that first passes through the birth canal (leading part) differs depending on the fetal position. In breech presentation, the hips, feet, and knees are the leading parts. Conversely, the scapula and hands become the advanced parts in the lateral position; however, the progress of labor stops.

Fetal presentation In the front-to-back and left-to-right orientations of the fetus in the uterus, the head and breech presentations show the relationship between the fetal back and the mother's body, and the lateral presentation shows the positional relationship between the fetal head and mother's body. A pattern in which the back or head faces the left side of the mother's body is referred to as the first fetal presentation, and a pattern in which the back or head faces the right side is referred to as the second fetal presentation.

Fetal attitude It represents the attitude of the fetus in the uterus and is classified into flexion and anti-bending. The normal fetal attitude is flexed, called parietal presentation, and the fetus is positioned as follows. Particularly, the head is strongly flexed forward, the chin touches the chest, and the spine is slightly flexed forward. The upper limbs are flexed at the elbows, the upper arms are close to the chest, and the forearms are crossed or parallel in front of the chest. The lower leg is strongly flexed at the knee and hip joints, and the thigh touches the abdomen. Legs are crossed or parallel, and the dorsum of the foot touches the lower leg. In this position, the fetus is oval with minimal volume and surface area. Conversely, the deflection position is divided into frontal, forehead, and face positions, depending on the degree.

Forceps delivery The fetus in this method of delivery is pulled out by grasping the fetal head from both sides with an instrument called forceps, which consists of two metal spatulas.

Vacuum extraction This delivery method occurs when a large round cup made of metal (hard cup) or silicone (soft cup) is applied to the fetal head, the air inside the cup is removed, and the suction force is used to pull the fetal head.

5 Sleeping Position

Lateral position Lateral is a position when the infant lies on their side. The position with the right side down is called the right lateral position, and the position with the left side down is called the left lateral position. It may be done when medically necessary, rather than in a position that the infant adopts on its own. The lateral position, along with the prone position, is associated with the risk of sudden infant death syndrome. The risk is reported to be particularly high if the infant is placed on the side while lying on their stomach (prone position).

Prone position (*Fukuga-i*) ⇒ lying on stomach

Supine position (*Gyoga-i*) ⇒ lying on back

Supine position (*Haiga-i*) ⇒ lying on back

Prone position Prone position is when the baby sleeps on their stomach with their face turned to the side in a natural manner. As prone position is a risk factor for sudden infant death syndrome (SIDS), infants should sleep on their backs (supine) until they are able to roll over.

Supine position Supine is a position when the infant lies on their back. In adults, the face is often turned upward, but is often turned to the left or right in early infancy.

Sudden infant death syndrome: SIDS This syndrome causes sudden death in infants aged <1 year, in which death cannot be predicted based on previous health conditions and medical history, and the cause of death cannot be identified by death scene investigation and autopsy examinations. Both prone and supine sleepers can develop SIDS; however, the incidence of SIDS is higher when lying prone. Since the "Back to Sleep" campaign to prevent SIDS in the United States, SIDS has declined; however, the incidence of plagiocephaly increased.

6 Prevention and Treatment of Positional Plagiocephaly

Aimet® Aimet® is a helmet for cranial shape correction manufactured and sold by the Japan Medical Company. Each helmet is made to order so that it can be corrected to the ideal head shape of Japanese infants. Under the supervision of a Japanese doctor, it received medical device approval (30100BZX00022000) in May 2019, was manufactured in Japan using a consistent process, and won the 2019 Good Design Award.

Cushion Cushion is a part that makes up a cranial shape correcting helmet and refers to the low-resilience sponge that is attached to the inside of the helmet. While dispersing the pressure by the cushion, it corrects by acting as a surface. It prevents pressure from concentrating on one point and reduces the risk of congestion.

Donut pillow A donut pillow is a baby pillow with a hollow or hole in the middle. This pillow has been used to prevent and treat positional cranial deformity; however, its scientific efficacy has not been fully demonstrated.

Fee for treatment of patients' choice Owing to the revision of medical fees in April 2016, a system was established by the Ministry of Health, Labour, and Welfare with the aim of promoting the division of functions and business collaboration among medical institutions, stating that "Early symptoms should be examined at local clinics and clinics, while advanced and specialized medical care should be provided at hospitals (with more than 200 beds)." When visiting a relatively large medical institution without a referral letter from a clinic, you will be required to pay an additional fee on top of the usual medical expenses.

Molded helmet therapy Helmet therapy is an intervention for infant cranial deformities of any cause. The purpose is to correct cranial deformity by wearing custom-made helmets for a long time. As of 2022, this treatment is not covered by health insurance.

Shell Officially called a helmet shell, this part makes up a cranial shape correction helmet. The shell is made using a 3D printer so that it can be guided to the ideal skull shape for each infant.

3D scanning 3D scanning is a method of photographing three-dimensional objects in various ways to capture them as 3D data. By attaching a sensor to the object or irradiating it with a laser beam, the 3D coordinate data of the object's "height (X)," "width (Y)," and "depth (Z)" can be obtained. Furthermore, a "point cloud data" is created by combining the coordinate data scanned from various angles. From there, it becomes 3D data by converting to "polygon data (mesh data)" covered with "triangular surfaces made by connecting coordinate points with straight lines." It becomes 3D data only after processing by using software after scanning. Together with the 3D printer described in the next section, 3D scanning is used to create corrective helmets.

3D printer 3D printers' layer cross-sectional shapes are based on 3D data created with 3D software such as 3D computer-aided design (CAD) and 3D CG (computer graphics). 3D printer is a general term for equipment that can be used for three-dimensional modeling.

Tummy time Tummy is "pom-pon" in baby talk (Japanese). The Japanese translation of tummy time has not been established by the Japanese Association of Medical Sciences. When an infant is awake, provide time for them to lie face down under the supervision of a parent or guardian. Japanese words, such as "utsubuse renshu (prone practice)," "harabai renshu (belly practice)," and "kubisuwari renshu (head practice)," are used. Recently, the term "utsubuse asobi (prone play)" has become commonly used.

7 Related to Academic Organizations

American Academy of Pediatrics (AAP) Founded in 1930, this organization is dedicated to optimizing the physical, mental, and social health and well-being of infants, children, adolescents, young adults, and pediatric health professionals who care for children. To date, AAP has 67,000 pediatricians, mainly in North America.

Japan Cranial Medical Examination and Treatment Society (JCMETS) JCMETS is a voluntary group that advocates for the "contribution to the progress and spread of cranial health check-ups and treatments by providing a forum for research communication, knowledge exchange, and collaboration between members and related academic organizations in Japan and abroad, and by contributing to the development of academic culture and the improvement of cranial medical examinations and treatments, we will contribute to the health and welfare of the people." It consists of doctors, midwives, nurses, and physical therapists.

MIX
Papier aus verantwortungsvollen Quellen
Paper from responsible sources
FSC® C105338

If you have any concerns about our products,
you can contact us on
ProductSafety@springernature.com

In case Publisher is established outside the EU,
the EU authorized representative is:
Springer Nature Customer Service Center GmbH
Europaplatz 3, 69115 Heidelberg, Germany

Printed by Libri Plureos GmbH
in Hamburg, Germany